Philosophy, Psychoanalysis, and the A-rational Mind

International Perspectives in Philosophy and Psychiatry

Series editors: Bill (K.W.M.) Fulford, Katherine Morris, John Z Sadler, and Giovanni Stanghellini

Volumes in the series:

Philosophy, Psychoanalysis, and the A-rational Mind

Linda A.W. Brakel
Departments of Philosophy & Psychiatry
The University of Michigan
Ann Arbobn, Michigan
U.S.A.

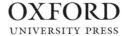

OXFORD
UNIVERSITY PRESS

OXFORD
UNIVERSITY PRESS

Great Clarendon Street, Oxford OX2 6DP

Oxford University Press is a department of the University of Oxford.
It furthers the University's objective of excellence in research, scholarship,
and education by publishing worldwide in

Oxford New York

Auckland Cape Town Dar es Salaam Hong Kong Karachi
Kuala Lumpur Madrid Melbourne Mexico City Nairobi
New Delhi Shanghai Taipei Toronto

With offices in

Argentina Austria Brazil Chile Czech Republic France Greece
Guatemala Hungary Italy Japan Poland Portugal

Oxford is a registered trade mark of Oxford University Press
in the UK and in certain other countries

Published in the United States
by Oxford University Press Inc., New York

British Library Cataloguing in Publication Data
Data available

Library of Congress Cataloguing in Publication Data
Data available

Typeset by Cepha Imaging Private Ltd., Bangalore, India
Printed in Great Britain
on acid-free paper by the MPG Books Group in the UK

ISBN 978–0–19–955125–5 (Pbk.)

10 9 8 7 6 5 4 3 2 1

To Arthur,
who makes it all worthwhile.

Permissions Granted

I thank the following publishing agencies, societies, and/or journals for their kind permission to publish in the present volume revised versions of works previously published. These are:

1. *The Psychoanalytic Quarterly* for "Book Review of *The Rediscovery of Mind* by John Searle" by Linda A.W. Brakel, which was first published in *The Psychoanalytic Quarterly*, 1994, Volume 62, pages 787–792, and here, in revised form, makes up part of Chapter 2.

2. Wiley-Blackwell for "On knowing the unconscious: lessons from the epistemology of geometry and space" by Linda A.W. Brakel, which originally was published in *The International Journal of Psychoanalysis*, 1994, Volume 75, pages 39–49, and here, in revised form contributes to Chapter 2.

3. Nicolaus Copernicus University Press for "Unusual human experiences: Kant, Freud, and an associationist law" by Linda A.W. Brakel, which was first published in *Theoria et Historia Scientiarum*, 2003, Volume 7, pages 109–119, and here, in revised form appears as Chapter 3.

4. *Journal of Evolutionary Psychology* for "The fate of the dream after awakening: stages toward analytic understanding" by Linda A.W. Brakel, which was first published in the *Journal of Evolutionary Psychology*, 1984, Volume 5, pages 97–108, and here, in revised form contributes to Chapter 4.

5. Taylor and Francis Ltd. Journals (http://www.informaworld.com) for "Phantasy and wish: a proper function account of a-rational primary process mediated mentation" by Linda A.W. Brakel, which was first published in *The Australasian Journal of Philosophy*, 2002, Volume 80, pages 1–16, and here, in revised form, appears as Chapter 5.

6. The Austrian Academy of Sciences (DOI: 10.1553/3-7001-3386-3s75) for "Drive theory and primary process: a philosophical account" by Linda A.W. Brakel. This first was published in Patrizia Giampieri-Deutsch (ed.): *Psychoanalysis as an Empirical, Interdisciplinary Science*, 2005, pages 75–90. Veroffentlichungen der Kommission fur Philosophice und Padagogik, Nr.27: Sitzungsberichte der philosphisch-historischen Klasse, 717. Wien. It now appears, in revised form, as Chapter 6.

7. *The American Journal of Psychoanalysis* for "Phantasies, neurotic-beliefs, and beliefs-proper" by Linda A.W. Brakel, originally published in *The American Journal of Psychoanalysis*, 2001, Volume 61, pages 363–389, and here, in revised form contributes to Chapter 7.

Preface

Aims

This book has four aims. First, it aims to demonstrate that psychoanalysis as a general theory of mind rests upon a core set of fundamental assumptions. It is from these foundational posits that the clinical psychoanalytic theory (in all of its versions) derives. Further, these foundational assumptions are sound, and place psychoanalysis within the framework of ordinary, normal scientific investigation.

Second, the book aims to explore in depth one of the assumptions—namely, that human mentation, in addition to our usual "rational," secondary process thought, consists in a different form of thought—primary process, "a-rational" mentation. Understanding a-rational primary process as having a separate formal organization, will provide grounds to reinvestigate several topics of interest to psychoanalysts, philosophers of mind and action, and academic psychologists studying cognition, affect and development—notably the cognitive and conative psychological attitudes, including wish, desire, phantasy, belief, and drive.

The third aim of the book follows from these investigations, as it will become clear that psychoanalytic concepts and clinical theories can and should be sharpened using the sort of rigor that philosophical analysis can supply.

The fourth aim is reciprocal to the third—philosophy of mind and action can likewise benefit as disciplines by having to take into account and explicate psychoanalytic data—data that has as much to do with thought that is unconscious and a-rational as with conscious and rational mentation.

Scope

Other books on these topics have of course been written. There are three in particular—*Irrationality and the Philosophy of Psychoanalysis* by Sebastian Gardner (1993); *Open Minded* by Jonathan Lear (1998); and *The Psychoanalytic Mind: From Freud to Philosophy* by Marcia Cavell (1993)—each of which I will deal with in a later chapter pointing out the contrasts. But as a preview, let me state what this current volume uniquely offers: (1) an account of psychoanalysis as a general theory of mind fitting in with ordinary science and requiring no special psychology (different from Gardner's view in which psychoanalysis is separate from Ordinary Psychology); (2) a coherent view of a-rationally medi-ated beliefs, desires, wishes, and even phantasies that are propositional (rather than the pre-propositional nature of phantasies for Gardner and Lear); and (3) an account of primary process a-rational mentation as developmentally earlier and not ontologically dependent upon secondary process (which differs from what Cavell holds).

Further, this book demonstrates the integrated use of psychoanalytic data, concepts, and theories with principles and concerns from the philosophy of mind and action, enriching both sides by constraining psychoanalytic theorizing, while broadening philosophy's scope. Thus, philosophers of mind and action, and psychoanalytic theorists, as well as clinical psychoanalysts (and clinical psychologists, psychiatrists, and social workers) might well find this book of value. At the same time it is hoped that academic psychologists of various stripes (e.g. developmental, cognitive, social) will also find this work of interest insofar as they too grapple with issues concerning the psychological attitudes, consciousness and unconscious mentation, rationality and its vicissitudes—topics directed toward understanding more fully the complex nature of the human mind.

Acknowledgments

I thank those at Oxford University Press (United Kingdom), particularly my editors, Martin Baum and Carol Maxwell, who have had a large role in helping this project take shape. For reviewing and commenting on earlier drafts of various chapters, I thank Andy Egan, Jim Joyce, Ruth Millikan, Jack Novick, Ian Proops, Peter Railton, and Tim Schroeder. Then there are three others, who while they too did review and comment on some of the chapters, did so much more. Therefore, I express my gratitude to Howard Shevrin, David Velleman, and especially my husband (and best friend and critic), Arthur Brakel.

Linda A.W. Brakel
Ann Arbor, Michigan
May, 2008

Contents

Part I

General considerations

Part I consists of Chapters 1 and 2. Chapter 1 introduces the conceptual foundations of psychoanalysis and then provides an outline of the structure of this book. Chapter 2 presents arguments against critics who challenge the very heart of this project; and then offers a positive account both for a-rational and unconscious, *contentful* mentation.

Chapter 1

Introduction

This book is about the philosophical implications of a set of important psycho-analytic concepts, all closely connected to the foundation of psychoanalytic theory. It examines selected intersections of philosophy and psychoanalysis, and it has two intersecting goals. One is to provide, through philosophical analyses, a level of conceptual rigor that has too often been lacking in address-ing psychoanalytic concepts. I hope the increased rigor will lead to a renewed appreciation for psychoanalytic theory as a general theory of mind. No less important is the second goal. Uniquely here, psychoanalytic topics are exam-ined philosophically with the aim of expanding philosophy's domain. Just as the philosophy of human action can embrace more than rationally mediated action, the philosophy of mind should extend to encompass more than rational and conscious mentation—the philosophy of mind can be a philosophy of the a-rational and unconscious mind too.

Although there are many important books about philosophy and psychoa-nalysis (e.g. Wisdom 1953; Wohlheim 1984; Edelson 1984, 1988; Lear 1990, 1998; Cavell 1993), this book is unusual in its applications of analyses from wide-ranging philosophical areas. There will be some use of philosophy of science, metaphysics, epistemology, as well as philosophy of mind, and philosophy of action—all singularly focused toward the better understanding of concepts closely connected with the *foundational structure of psychoanalysis as a general theory of mind.* Indeed, despite the complexity of psychoanalytic clinical theory, and the recent proliferation of different psychoanalytic "schools" purportedly underwritten by different aspects of the clinical theory, the essential features of any and every branch of psychoanalysis can be derived from the several basic assumptions comprising the general psychoanalytic theory of mind.[1] Thus, before embarking on the philosophical investigation of

---

[1] According to Wallerstein (2005a) different psychoanalytic schools have existed at least since the 1920s. By the last quarter of the twentieth century, in addition to that which had been considered the standard version—retaining and extending Freud's views—and best described as ego psychology/conflict and compromise, one could count four schools. These included Kleinian, Lacanian, British object relations, and self-psychology psychoanalysis.

the particular concepts to be taken up in the chapters of this book, I now turn to the vital task of this introduction—presenting the foundational structure of psychoanalysis as a general theory of mind. It is a general theory both simple and elegant, consisting of just five fundaments.

The foundational structure of psychoanalysis

Psychoanalysis, like any scientific theory, has a small number of necessary basic underlying presuppositions. As is the case for all such assumptions, these fundamental postulates are (1) taken for granted, (2) used to derive other psychoanalytic propositions and concepts, and when functioning (3) generate psychoanalytic data.[2] In my view (and consequently the view held throughout this book) three assumptions, one methodological tool, and one corollary

Subsequently, in the last decade or so another school rose to prominence—relational psychoanalysis; and along with this several sub-schools—the social constructivists, the interpersonal, and the intersubjective.

I should point out that my view—that all branches of psychoanalysis share the general theory—is not a universally held one. Wallerstein (1988, 1990), for example, who is widely known in the psychoanalytic world for his position that there is a "common ground" among all the psychoanalytic schools, asserts that the essential commonality owes to psychoanalytic *clinical theory*, not the *general theory*. But Wallerstein (2005a, p. 624) recognizes that his notion of the common ground is far from generally accepted; he alludes to "a chorus of critics" who claim that different metapsychologies necessarily lead to different clinical theories and techniques. Here I adhere to the arguments of the critics, but with an important addition—if the different metapsychologies do not include the five basic fundaments of psychoanalytic general theory, they are not psychoanalytic theories, whether or not the clinical theories and techniques give the impression of psychoanalytic common ground. (For more on this topic see Shevrin *et al.*, 1996, chapter 2.)

[2] Psychoanalytic data broadly include everything reported and taking place in psychoanalytic sessions—for example, dream contents; psychological symptoms such as phobias, obsessions, excessive anxiety, and depressive mood; sexual concerns; slips of the tongue and parapraxes (mistakes in action); phantasies and daydreams; and reports of strong feelings about persons past and present, including the analyst. Although such psychoanalytic data can indeed demonstrate the plausibility, coherence, and explanatory value of the initial assumptions, evidence for these foundational postulates cannot be gained using these data insofar as they presume the very assumptions in question. (See Freud 1915b; Edelson 1984; Shevrin 1984; Brakel 1991; Shevrin *et al.*, 1996.) For this reason, the research I participate in as an Associate Director of the Hunt Memorial Laboratory at the University of Michigan (directed by Howard Shevrin) is devoted to testing psychoanalytic assumptions with data generated by methods *independent* of psychoanalytic assumptions. Such convergent evidence *can* contribute to assessing the validity of the basic psychoanalytic assumptions.

comprise the entire foundational core of psychoanalysis as a *general* theory of mind.[3]

The first two assumptions, psychic (psychological) continuity and psychic (psychological) determinism are best considered together. They are psychology-specific versions of two general assumptions that are in place given any scientific theory. Continuity presumes some sort of regularity or lawfulness in the phenomena under study,[4] and determinism means simply that the operation of cause and effect is presumed. To assume *psychic continuity* then is to take for granted that all of any agent's psychological events—including those that look inconsistent or even incoherent such as pathological symptoms (for instance, phobias to water, benign animals or of open places), slips of the tongue, and parapraxes—are regular/lawful in a particular *psychological* way for that agent; namely that every psychological event can be understood as *psychologically meaningful* to that individual. Similarly, to assume *psychic determinism* is to presume that all psychological events—even those that look incoherent—have at least as one of their causes, a *psychological cause*, and can thereby be explained (at least in part) on a psychological basis. So for example, a dream element, a delusion, a confabulation all can be presumed to be necessarily regular and lawful phenomena with physical and psychological causes such that these phenomena cannot fail to be psychologically meaningful to the dreaming, delusional, or confabulating agent. Put another way, there is no dream element, delusion, or confabulation, in fact no psychological content possible for a particular person that will not have been caused by some aspect of that person's psychology and that will not thereby be meaningful to that person.

---

[3] My view in the present work owes much to, but alters and elaborates that of Freud (1900, 1915b), Rapaport (1944), Shevrin (1984), Brakel (1991), and Shevrin (*et al.*, 1996). Each of these authors has picked out concepts as foundational so as to bring order to the unruly entity called "psychoanalytic theory." I continue in this tradition, claiming only that my selection, pertaining just to the general theory, is simpler. For example, Rapaport, although acknowledging that clinical psychoanalytic theory is distinct from the general theory, nonetheless considers "carry[ing] the method of interpersonal relationship to its last consequences (p. 202)" as one of the basic assumptions. For me, while this is indeed a central element for any account of psychoanalytic technique, it is part of the clinical, not the general theory. Parallel to my attempt here to derive the general theory from basic foundational concepts, Rubenstein (1976) proposes the fundaments for a strictly clinical psychoanalytic theory.

[4] The type of regularity and lawfulness is not tightly constrained. But some regularity/lawfulness, however minimal, is needed to even allow any scientific investigation to get underway—for example, to be capable of picking out particular phenomena as the phenomena to study.

For instance, suppose I have a physiologic derangement that causes me to have delusions. The content of each particular delusion I have must be psychologically caused and psychologically meaningful to me. Suppose now that you have the same physiologic condition and even the same delusional content. Still the psychological cause and psychological meaning of that identical content for you will uniquely be a function of your psychological continuity and determination, not mine.

The third assumption of psychoanalysis is that there exists a *dynamic* (*psychologically meaningful*) *unconscious*. It is posited because without such a postulate many psychological events "seem" neither psychically continuous nor determined. Take a very common sort of slip of the tongue I experienced. I was in the backyard calling my husband whom I saw to be occupied with some yard activity. He did not respond, a fact that did not surprise me as much as the realization that I was using our dog's name to call him, not my husband's. I laughed. Now, the names Art and Jet are not dissimilar—and that was a physical cause of the slip; but why would I (a neurologically intact person) confuse my husband's name with that of our dog's? This slip of the tongue seems neither psychologically lawful nor determined *until* we posit a dynamic unconscious cause of this commonplace psychological event. My husband, whom I love, seemed to me as unresponsive as our dog, a canine whom I also love. I was unconsciously angry with him; and unconsciously, but ambivalently, I insulted him—you are no better than our (wonderful, albeit very disobedient) dog. As with this simple example, the assumption of interceding unconscious processes and contents allows psychological determinism and continuity to be evident generally, even in those psychological events (such as neurotic symptoms, dream elements, delusions, and hallucinations) seemingly inconsistent to the point of frank bizarreness.

The one methodological tool necessary for psychoanalysis is *free association*. Free association as part of the foundational core of psychoanalytic general theory has an interesting status in that it functions in a dual manner. First, free associations demonstrate apparent violations of psychic continuity and psychic determinism by revealing psychological events like parapraxes and symptoms that seem incoherent, with no meaningful psychological cause. Second, free associations resolve the apparent violations in continuity and determinism by providing the psychological contents, which when taken in conjunction with the assumption of a dynamic unconscious, can render what was seemingly inconsistent as quite continuous, now admitting of transparent psychological causation.

Here is an example of the dual functioning of free association. A patient under analysis expressed anger at me for "going on vacation so much and 'cancering' her sessions." Her slip of the tongue occurred as she freely associated; this speech parapraxis was a psychological event that seemed discontinuous. But, by assuming psychic continuity, psychic determinism, and a dynamic unconscious, we can however hold that there was a psychologically relevant set of unconscious contents causing this particular slip, and further, that if the patient could continue to free associate, including associating to her slip of the tongue, its causal contents could be revealed. My patient did associate to her parapraxis: *she talked, as she often had, of fearing that I would go off, have a baby, and abandon her. She had never had a thought about my having cancer. She continued that her mother had been sick during her pregnancy with her younger sibling and therefore not very attentive to her; and that after he was born it was even worse, she really felt abandoned. She thought she probably hated her newborn brother and her mother.* These free associations revealed the unconscious contents that likely caused the seemingly discontinuous event and restored continuity. The patient feared something inside me would grow and take me away from her. Consciously, whenever I went on vacations she worried that the past would be repeated—that I would leave her by becoming pregnant and she would feel abandoned. Unconsciously, whenever I went on vacation she was so angry with me for leaving her that she wished me to be sick with a growing cancer instead of a growing baby.

The final element comprising the foundational structure of psychoanalytic general theory—positing *primary and secondary processes* as two formally different types of mentation—is best described as a corollary to the other fundaments. The corollary status obtains because positing primary and secondary processes follows from and is demonstrated by the application of the three basic assumptions and free association.[5] The primary and secondary processes operating according to different principles can, for instance, be appreciated in the above examples. Secondary process thinking is the largely rational, rule-following, ordinary logic of adults in the alert, waking state. Primary process thinking, in contrast, is a-rational[6] and associatively based.

---

[5] As is true for the assumptions of psychoanalysis, gaining evidence for the corollary—the existence of primary and secondary process mentation—also requires data and methods independent of psychoanalytic presuppositions. (For more on independent evidence see Shevrin *et al.*, 1996. For examples of such independent evidence for the existence of primary and secondary process mentation see Brakel, 2004; Brakel *et al.*, 2002; Brakel and Shevrin 2005.)

[6] I use the term "a-rational" quite deliberately. "A-rationality" is much broader in its application than is "irrationality," the term more typically employed. Whereas irrationality implies rationality that has gone astray, entailing a dispositional capacity for rationality,

When the secondary processes predominate, psychological events look continuous, caused, explainable, and rational. Thus, if I had been thinking at a secondary process, level I would have called out my husband's name since I had wanted him to respond. Similarly, if my patient's functioning had been predominately secondary process, she might have directly experienced her anger at me for taking a vacation in the midst of her psychoanalytic work and even recognized that the strength of her feeling abandoned owed to her distant past. Primary process thinking, on the other hand, is clearly not rational. Instead, it is a-rational. It is the type of mentation operative when I categorized my husband-who-does-not-respond with our disobedient dog, and displaced his name with her's. Likewise, when my patient spoke of my "cancering" the sessions she demonstrated a primary process type of categorization. Tumors and babies are both things that grow inside and take mother figures away. Because my leaving on vacation felt like abandonment, she was angry and displaced the baby she feared I would have with a tumor she wished I would have.

Primary process thinking is a-rational thinking. Its hallmarks, in addition to the absence of ordinary rationality, displacement, and the type of feature-based categorizing by resemblance shown above, include condensations (combining thoughts that by ordinary logic do not belong together), categorizations by contiguity in time and/or space, and substitutions of part for whole. Dream elements perhaps provide the most obvious, plentiful, and accessible examples of primary process contents demonstrating the effects of the operation (in all combinations) of these many a-rational primary processes.

Organizational plan of the book

The fundamental postulates of psychoanalysis as a general scientific theory of mind[7] consist of three assumptions—psychic continuity, psychic

---

a-rationality implies no such thing. Thinking, for example, can be a-rational if it is "not-yet-rational" as in very young humans and "never-to-be-rational/but good enough for survival" as in certain birds and mammals. (See Brakel 2002; Brakel and Shevrin 2003.) That for Freud the primary processes were developmentally earlier suggests that even on a standard psychoanalytic account, a-rationality more properly describes the primary process mode of thinking. Note that the a-rational primary processes are very frequently appropriated to irrational ends as is evidenced in most psychological symptoms. (Indeed this might be the source of the mischaracterization of the primary processes as irrational instead of a-rational.)

[7] Popper (1963) held that psychoanalytic theory is not falsifiable and hence not even a potentially scientific theory. There are also many within psychoanalysis, who for reasons

determinism, a dynamic unconscious; one methodological tool—free association; and one corollary—that primary as well as secondary process mentation exists. This view of the foundational core of the general psychoanalytic theory of mind provides the background for the book. The assumptions of psychic continuity and psychic determinism (assumptions one and two, respectively), the most basic of the fundaments and grounds for all else in psychoanalytic theory, will remain very much in the background. Instead this book will focus directly one level down on assumption three—the existence of a dynamic meaningful (contentful) unconscious; and corollary one—positing two different forms of thought, the primary and secondary processes. In each chapter particular philosophical analyses are applied to one or both of these foundational elements, and/or to concepts readily derived from them, in order to make good on the book's dual motivating claims that the philosophical analyses can provide the conceptual rigor that has been lacking in psychoanalytic theory; and that psychoanalytic topics, when examined philosophically, can expand philosophy's domain.

The book is organized into five parts and will consist of ten chapters.

Part I: General considerations

In addition to Chapter 1, "Introduction," this part will include Chapter 2, titled "Just what sort of theory is psychoanalytic theory?" This chapter deals with two specific problems with psychoanalytic theory: (1) that it posits (from assumption three) unconscious mentation, and (2) that it presupposes (from corollary one) mentation organized according to principles different from those organizing ordinary adult thought—the form of thought Freud (1895, 1900, 1915b, 1940) called primary process. These are problems requiring philosophy of science, metaphysical, and epistemological attention. However, skeptics

---

different from Popper's, claim that psychoanalytic theory is not a scientific theory. Indeed there is a sizeable literature on the debate itself. However, this matter will not be addressed here. I have taken as starting point for this book that psychoanalysis *is* a scientific theory. (Nonetheless, for a sense of this controversy within psychoanalytic circles see Shevrin's, 1995, article, "Is Psychoanalysis One Science, Two Sciences, or No Science at all?" first delivered as a plenary address to the American Psychoanalytic Association in 1993, and published two years later with a series of commentaries on the conflictual issues.)

Similarly, problems with free association as the methodologically necessary tool for psychoanalysis are not taken up. This, despite the fact that critics, most vociferously Grunbaum (1984), have argued that suggestion, not free association is the vehicle of psychoanalytic change.

who challenge the existence of unconscious representations present a pressing prior concern—namely they question the very conceptualization of contentful unconscious mentation. Because this position threatens the entire project at its base, the work of Chapter 2 begins by addressing two such critics of unconscious representation, each coming from a very different perspective—first the philosopher John Searle (1992), and then the cognitive scientists, Pierre Perruchet and Annie Vinter (2002).

After defending psychoanalytic general theory against these skeptical critics, the task of Chapter 2 is to launch the positive project. I begin by presenting the standard psychoanalytic presuppositions regarding (1) unconscious mentation and (2) the nature of the primary processes. Owing to convention (if not definition) ordinary thought has been widely regarded as necessarily both conscious and rational. Thus, the unconscious type of mentation, and the primary process mediated type of a-rational thought, both posited by and essential to psychoanalytic theory, must be considered outside-the-ordinary forms of thought. The very possibility of outside-the-ordinary forms of thought opens the way to arguing that the problems in positing unconscious and primary process thought are deeply analogous with certain Kantian ontologic and epistemologic problems. For Kant, the possibility of any content outside-the-categories is problematic—the categories necessary for understanding entail that whatever can be understood and experienced must be within-the-categories (Kant 1781, 1787). By specifically offering outside-the-categories solutions acceptable to philosophers of science regarding problems in theories of the geometry of space—an area that has classically presented ontologic and epistemologic difficulties for Kantians—a model is proposed for solving the analogous and surprisingly similar problems with the psychoanalytic theory of unconscious and primary process mentation.

Part II: Epistemological issues

This part more directly concerns epistemology and will investigate Freudian primary process (corollary one) and secondary process in Kantian terms. Chapter 3, "Did Kant precede Freud on a-rational thought?," examines a little heralded primary process precursor in Kant's ontology of thinking (Kant 1783).

Chapter 4, "Why primary process mentation is hard to know," explores a powerful force—the force with which ordinary, secondary process, within-the-categories, mostly rational thought strives to reorganize primary process manifestations in order to experience them as ordinary and mostly rational. Using dreams and their contents as common and familiar examples of primary process mentation, I describe dream formation and the fate of the dream after awakening. In Chapter 4, I suggest that dreams proceed in stages, early on consisting in primary process content outside Kant's categories, but eventually conforming to secondary process content fully determined by the categories. Dreams are (1) first dreamt, (2) subsequently remembered, (3) and finally rehearsed to oneself to recount to another (the analyst).

Part III: Something new for the philosophy of mind

This part consists entirely in Chapter 5, "Representational a-rational thinking: A proper function account," the heart of my project. Here I make the claim that primary process mentation (corollary one)—essentially a-rational rather than rational—is nonetheless a truly representational system of thought. The most prevalent view in the philosophy of mind is that for a mental state to be contentful it must be part of a holistically rational system of beliefs and desires. This allows and necessitates that successful interpretation of a mental state based on rational normativity constitutes and "fixes" the determinate (and usually singularly determined) content of the mental state. An example will make this much clearer. Suppose (as is actually the case) that every autumn Ann Arbor becomes a college football crazed town. Suppose further that it is a football Saturday. In this context imagine that two people are having a conversation about the arrival today of A's in-laws in Ann Arbor to see the big home game. Person B then says something about his own mother-in-law, namely that she is a big Michigan football fan. When A replies that as far as he is concerned he hopes that the visitors get killed today, it is entirely clear that he is not talking about his in-laws but about some visiting football team. It is assumed that A is largely rational and that his communications will reflect largely rational beliefs and desires. Expressing casually one's hopes for the death of one's in-laws is not rational. Thus what might have been indeterminate content regarding "visitors getting killed" is fixed and determinate in line with successfully interpreting Person A as having (1) the rational belief that a visiting football team is coming to town, and (2) the rational desire that this team be defeated.[8]

Meanwhile, no part of this formula for determining and fixing content—assuming holistic rationality, then using rational normativity to successfully

---

[8] Note that from a psychoanalytic perspective, it may be the case that Person A is also expressing an unconscious death wish toward his in-laws. Content that is not singularly determinate need not be indeterminate. This matter will be addressed directly in Chapter 6.

interpret particular beliefs and desires—will work for a-rational mentation. A-rational mentation is neither rational nor in the standard belief/desire form. Thus in this chapter another way to deal with the threat of indeterminacy must be proposed, and it is. Primary process mental states, I argue, can gain sufficient determinacy of content via a proper function naturalistic account. Here evolutionary success and selective fitness normativity, instead of interpretative success and rational normativity, determine and constitute the content of particular mental states. In this way, independent both of rationality and the view of interpreters, primary process mentation can be shown to be contentful.

But the case for this view requires something further—a viable proper function account for primary process mentation—in other words, an argument for the view that the primary processes, when functioning properly, enhance the selective fitness success of those using primary process mentation. Toward the end of Chapter 5, I offer such an account, intrinsic to which is the view that properly functioning primary processes take the form of phantasy and wish rather than belief and desire. The causal role of such primary process phantasies and wishes in many psychological acts demonstrates limitations in the standard belief/desire propositional attitude psychology favored by philosophers to explain motivation and intention.

Part IV: A philosophy of action view of psychoanalysis

Discovering limitations in standard belief/desire psychology accounts of motivation and intention provide a bridge to this part. Chapter 6, "Psychoanalytic drives,"deals with the philosophical analysis of drives and, particularly, the non-singular, primary process (corollary one) nature of drive objects. Within this chapter a distinction between indeterminate and not singularly determinate is taken up with reference to the philosophical issue of vagueness. I argue that primary process concepts, despite superficial appearances, are not vague concepts.

Chapter 7, "Phantasies, beliefs, and neurotic-beliefs," and Chapter 8, "Desires and the readiness to act," the two most clinical chapters, also deal with inadequacies in belief/desire explanations of human action, particularly as unconscious aspects (assumption three) are not considered. Both chapters present the consequences of confusions of one sort of psychological attitude for another. Chapter 7 makes the case that "neurotic-beliefs," while actually having the structure of unconscious phantasies, are experienced by the (neurotic-) believers as conscious beliefs and treated as though they have the same causal role as beliefs. Chapter 8 argues for "the readiness to act" as the constitutive function of desire—both unconscious and conscious desire—and highlights troubles when desires are seen as merely unacceptable wishes.

Part V: Conclusions and summary

This part consists of two chapters. Chapter 9, "Compare and contrast," offers a brief look at the views of Sebastian Gardner in *Irrationality and the Philosophy of Psychoanalysis*, Jonathan Lear in *Open Minded*, and Marcia Cavell in *The Psychoanalytic Mind*, to evaluate the similarities and differences with respect to the views presented in this book. As will be no surprise, I argue for the advantages provided by the accounts herein.

In Chapter 10, "Conclusions and summary," I restate and repeat my evidence for the opening claim that philosophical analyses of psychoanalytic theory can be of benefit both to philosophy and psychoanalysis. Psychoanalytic theory, I claim, stands to gain by incorporating the rigor of philosophical analyses, while it is of benefit to the philosophy of mind and the philosophy of action to extend their domains. Examples from the body of the book will be cited, reviewing many of the volume's other major points as the validity of this claim is demonstrated. The final emphasis suggests that by providing an open passageway between the psychoanalytic general theory of mind and the philosophies of mind and action, this book points the way toward a welcome sea change in both disciplines. Psychoanalytic theory, if it is to be considered seriously, can and should become more sharply defined. The philosophy of mind (and action), in order to encompass the more complete mind, can and should expand beyond the narrow confines of the conscious and rational to become the philosophy of the unconscious and a-rational mind as well.

Chapter 2

Just what sort of theory is psychoanalytic theory?

The psychoanalytic theory of mind is unique among general theories of mind in two ways: it assumes that (1) unconscious mentation is centrally important, and (2) that a nonrational mode of thinking—primary process mentation— plays a large role in most, if not all, psychological events. These two unique features, while unproblematic for the psychoanalyst who has embraced the theory, are highly contested in the academy both by philosophers of mind and cognitive psychologists because theories of mind have largely been theories of the conscious and rational mind. Thus from the viewpoint of philosophers of mind and cognitive psychologists, the psychoanalytic general theory of mind faces two immediate and serious problems.

First, psychoanalytic theory as a general theory of mind posits *unconscious* mentation as a core feature of mental functioning.[1] This includes both unconscious mental processes and unconscious mental contents. Unconscious mental processes include psychological defensive operations, as well as categorization, generalization, differentiation, and induction processes. Unconscious mental contents are unconscious representations *of* various items, ideas, and states. Here the operative word is "of" in that an unconscious content or representation must be "about" something, just as is true for a conscious content.

Second, psychoanalytic theory presumes, in addition to rationally mediated adult cognition, the existence of *primary process* cognition. This is a type of mentation organized according to principles different from those organizing ordinary *secondary process* adult thought. The primary processes are most readily appreciated in psychological events in which their influence is obvious— for example, our nightly dreams. The dreams we dream and then remember are rife with elements that are organized in a primary process fashion. Take, for instance, a dream of mine in which a colleague named Bob Hatcher behaved just like my mother. On awakening I could not understand this; these two

---

[1] The terms "mental" and "psychological" are for the most part interchangeable.

people did not seem at all alike—not in terms of any rational or logical category. I then suddenly realized that since I do have a brother named Robert, my mother is indeed a Robert-hatcher. The organizing principles forming the dream element (and understanding it) are associative, cross modal, nonlogical— they are instead a-rational, neither logical nor rational. Thus, Robert Hatcher and my mother form a primary process category on the basis of an inessential feature—his name (Robert Hatcher) and one of her functions (the hatcher of Robert). No such category arises using the criteria of secondary process organizing principles, those operative in everyday rational thought. In secondary process terms, Robert Hatcher is a name representing a person, not any sort of hatching activity, and the behaviors of the two people, Bob Hatcher and my mother, are compared according to a number of rational criteria.

This chapter will address the problems psychoanalytic general theory faces— those regarding unconscious processes and representations, and concerning the primary processes. But first, since positing meaningful unconscious processes and representations is the necessary core of any psychoanalytic theory of mind, skeptics who challenge the very conceptualization of unconscious mental content and processes must be answered—this before any positive account of the nature of the psychoanalytic theory of mind can be given. In this chapter two such skeptical positions will be discussed, one from the philosophy of mind and the other from cognitive science. They were chosen as emblematic, and particularly cogent and articulate representatives, of a large group of theorists who find the notion of the psychoanalytic unconscious either wrong or unnecessary.[2] First there is the view of philosopher John Searle (1992), who while allowing that repression (and other processes involved in transforming and disguising content) exists, claims that nonetheless what is unconscious cannot be contentful, that is, representational, *about* something, meaningful and intentional; instead it can only have "as-if" (or pseudo) intentionality—by which Searle means intentionality derived from conscious content. And then there is the position of Pierre Perruchet and Annie Vinter (2002), cognitive scientists arguing from parsimony that the concept of unconscious representations is not necessary. Interestingly, both Searle, and Perruchet and Vinter also

---

[2] I am not attempting an exhaustive review of arguments against the unconscious. Rather, insofar as Searle's view and that of Perruchet and Vinter are representative of many in philosophy of mind and cognitive science who dismiss the concept of a meaningful unconscious, my goal is more circumscribed. Namely, my aim is to demonstrate that even these highly esteemed, widely disseminated accounts of the impossibility or the nonnecessity of unconscious representational thought are quite flawed.

argue against the primary processes as being mental or psychological. Let us take a look at the Searle challenge first.

Answering skeptics

Searle[3]

In *The Rediscovery of Mind* (1992), an important work in the philosophy of mind, Searle has a good deal to say about the unconscious. This is especially so in Chapter 7, "The unconscious and its relation to consciousness." Much of what Searle says in this chapter is uncontroversial, no matter what view one holds on the ontology of unconscious representations. Regarding consciousness, Searle holds that it consists of conscious mental states that are not only first person and subjective, but necessarily *about* something. This *aboutness* is called intentionality. A bit more problematic, Searle goes on to characterize the unconscious in the following way: "the ontology of the unconscious is strictly the ontology of a neurophysiology capable of generating the conscious" (p. 172). Those holding the view that unconscious representations do exist need to take issue here, but only with the word "strictly," as Searle's dispositional account of the unconscious—the unconscious is that collection of neurophysiological processes disposed to causing what was merely potentially conscious to be conscious—is quite consistent with, although in no way a sufficient or complete account of, the classic psychoanalytic concept of repression. In the psychoanalytic account what has been repressed is *disposed* to become conscious or at least exert active influence on what does become conscious. And indeed Searle has no problem with certain unconscious desires and beliefs, those he terms "Freudian cases ... of repressed consciousness ... always bubbling to the surface, though often in disguised form" (pp. 172–3).[4] But the agreement between Searle and psychoanalytic theorists ends with Searle's assertion that the Freudian position (and the one held in this book) is incoherent—namely that unconscious mental states exist not merely dispositionally, but as mental, subjective, and *intentional* states even while unconscious. Searle states (p. 168) that "Freud thinks that our unconscious mental states exist both as unconscious and as occurrent intrinsic

---

[3] Much of what follows in this section appears in Brakel (1994b), a book review essay of *The Rediscovery of Mind*. This review appears in the *Psychoanalytic Quarterly* Vol. 63: 788–90.

[4] The transforming processes disguising these contents are the primary processes; here it seems that Searle allows these as mental.

intentional states even when their ontology is that of the mental, even when they are unconscious.[5] Can he [Freud] make such a picture coherent?" A bit later (Ibid., p. 168) Searle answers, "I cannot find or invent a coherent interpretation of this theory." But the assumption of unconscious contents and processes about subjectively meaningful matters (assumption three) is a vital and indeed a necessary assumption for psychoanalysis.

The crux of the disagreement turns on the understanding of "mental." Thus, whereas Searle sees "true ascriptions of unconscious mental life as corresponding to an objective neurophysiological ontology, but described in terms of its capacity to cause conscious subjective mental phenomena" (p. 168), he is troubled by the view that "Their ontology [that of unconscious mental states] is that of the mental, even when they are unconscious" (p. 168). This is the discomfort motivating his dispositional-only view of unconscious content. And yet the source of Searle's discomfort does not seem warranted, as the psychoanalytic view of unconscious mental states fits perfectly Searle's own definitional description of the ontology of mental phenomena. For Searle mental phenomena, which for him are conscious mental phenomena, are simply "caused by neurophysiological processes in the brain and are themselves features of the brain" (p. 1). It is in fact hard to see how any version of a representational unconscious mental state would fail to meet these criteria.

What does resolve the dilemma of Searle's need for his dispositional-only view of unconscious mental states is this: it is apparent that *Searle essentially requires consciousness to be a necessary feature of the mental.* Thus if consciousness is an ontologic criterion for being mental, *by definition* nothing unconscious can be mental.

Related to this matter, Searle holds that associations need not have any underlying "mental" process. He makes a distinction between rule-following

---

[5] Note that Galen Strawson (1994) defends a position more extreme than Searle's—in effect reducing the distance between Searle's view and that of psychoanalysis. For Strawson, what is mental must be mentally contentful and experienced now (p.168). On Searle's (1992) account *nonoccurrent, dispositional* beliefs, desires, intentions, and so on, even unconscious ones (e.g. I have a belief that snow is white and an intention to go to Australia, neither of which I am experiencing now, but both of which I have experienced in the past and will experience later) are contentful, intentional (about something), and mental, not withstanding the fact that the ontology of the mental is strictly neurophysiologic (Searle 1992, pp. 158–9). This is the case insofar as these are all "in principle accessible to consciousness" (p. 159). For Strawson (1994, p.168), Searle's view is highly problematic; no less so than the psychoanalytic position on unconscious beliefs, phantasies, desires, and wishes, in which these mental states are held to be *non-experiential and yet occurrent*, mental, contentful, and intentional, again with a strictly neurophysiologic ontology.

processes, which are mental (and intentional), and associations such as those via resemblance (and presumably via the other primary process/associative principles: contiguity in time or space, part for whole, etc.), "which need not have any mental content at all in addition to that of relata" (p. 240). Thus notwithstanding his earlier allusion to disguised repressed contents returning to consciousness, thereby implying the existence of transforming processes effecting these disguises (pp. 172–3), he warns that any ascription of mental content to such associational processes would be like ascribing mental content to the brute fixed nonconscious brain processes underlying visual experience (p. 240). For Searle, mental content ascription in either case would be a serious error, as both nonconscious visual processing and associational phenomena cannot have genuine intentionality, but only "as-if" (pseudo) intentionality parasitic upon the intentionality of rule-following mental operations. Thus and again *by definition, Searle has also excluded primary process operations from the mental.*

By-definition claims and counterclaims are usually stalemates, but Searle in making room for both repression and disguise provides an opening for counterarguments to his position that the ontology of the mental must include only conscious secondary process mediated states. He asserts:

> The ontology of the unconscious consists in objective features of the brain capable of causing subjective conscious thoughts [Searle's italics].... But the existence of these causal features is consistent with the fact that in any given case their causal powers may be blocked by some other interfering causes, such as psychological repression. (1992, p. 160)

By granting this, along with acknowledging that repressed desires and beliefs are always "bubbling to the surface … often in disguised form" (pp. 172–3), Searle has allowed opponents to his limited ontology of the mental to gain ground simply by asking a few questions naturally following Searle's view. Just how would Searle account for the "psychological repression" or the "disguising"? Wouldn't some truly mental, intentional, personal assessment be required, even though unconscious, to recognize that some sort of repression or disguise or other defense is needed? After all, the repressing as well as that which is repressed remain totally unconscious. And what about those transforming processes, not accessible to consciousness, yet resulting in the sort of disguise that can only be characterized as highly subjectively relevant—wouldn't these too best (even necessarily) be considered mental, intentional, and subjective?[6]

---

[6] Here are two examples, one illustrating the intentionality entailed by repressing a specific statement and the other the intentionality entailed when a transforming process disguises a particular content. Imagine a man, R, who desires an illicit relationship with his neighbor, a lovely, intelligent woman, W. He does not act on this desire for two reasons—(1) he

Perruchet and Vinter

While not overtly skeptical about unconscious representations, the cognitive scientists Perruchet and Vinter (2002) wrote a target piece, "The Self-organizing Consciousness," for *Behavioral and Brain Sciences*, that offers a theory of self-organizing consciousness (SOC) as a mentalistic framework they claim to be *sufficient* to explain all psychological phenomena *without positing unconscious representations*. Arguing against a "cognitive framework [that] rests on the existence of a powerful cognitive unconscious ... and the possibility of performing manipulations and transformations of unconscious representations" (p. 297), Perruchet and Vinter describe their SOC theory:

> We propose that the isomorphism generally observed in the world between the representations composing our momentary phenomenal experience and the structure of the world is the end-product of a progressive organization that emerges thanks to elementary associative processes that take our conscious representations themselves as the stuff on which they operate ... [This is our] ... concept of Self-Organizing Consciousness (SOC). (p. 297)

Clearly in Perruchet and Vinter's SOC model no unconscious representations are presumed. This is important as Perruchet and Vinter oppose their theory of mental organization directly to theories that do presuppose both unconscious representations and unconscious mental processes acting upon them. Since it is an accepted philosophy of science convention that in the absence of better explanations and predictions from one of two competing theories, the more parsimonious one, the one with the fewest posits, is to be preferred, Perruchet and Vinter's claim is of major theoretical interest.

Because the argument from parsimony demands only that Perruchet and Vinter demonstrate that their mentalistic framework *can* be sufficient to explain all relevant psychological phenomena, they need not establish that

fears W's husband, (2) he knows adultery would be harmful to his own marriage and her's. One day in casual conversation W's husband tells R, "I'll be away for the entire day on Wednesday." On Thursday, R suddenly remembers that he missed his chance; he had thought on Wednesday of visiting W, but told himself that another day would be just as good. R repressed the fact of W's husband's absence. Take another man, D, in the very same circumstances—desiring an illicit relationship with W, and learning from W's husband that he will be away on Wednesday. D on Wednesday thinks of visiting his neighbor W, but then "remembers" she is out of town. D unconsciously distorted the facts, disguising the fact that it was W's husband who would be absent. That neither man, R or D, acted on his conflicted desires owed in part to unconscious defensive operations, operations applied totally unconsciously but specifically and intentionally to subjectively meaningful content.

inferring unconscious representations is necessarily in error. Thus, seemingly the only ways to refute Perruchet and Vinter would be to show that their SOC is either not sufficient to account for particular psychological phenomena of interest or not generalizable enough to account for important basic psychological operations. These arguments can be made and were in fact made by many of the commentators on this target article.[7] I however will take another tack. While Perruchet and Vinter claim that their SOC without unconscious representations is a more parsimonious theory of the mental framework, I will claim that it is more parsimonious only superficially—while in deeper, more vital respects their theory is actually less parsimonious and precisely because it does not posit unconscious representations.

In my view the Perruchet and Vinter mentalistic framework, featuring only the readily obvious conscious representations, compared to a theory with unconscious representations inferred, is analogous to Ptolemy's astronomy, featuring the readily observed rotation of the sun about the earth, compared to the Copernican alternative that required an inferential leap. Ptolemy's theory required multiple conceptual additions (the epicycles) to remain accurate to the facts, but these reduced its elegance considerably. Four interlocking matters will demonstrate that Perruchet and Vinter's SOC theory, a theory without unconscious representations, likewise requires several burdensome corrections to make it operational—corrections not needed for theories of mind that include unconscious representations.

First, Perruchet and Vinter make the claim that unconscious representations have no functional role. If this claim is holds, it would provide powerful support for their view that unconscious representations are not necessary. But they do not make their case. They begin their argument by stating that revered scholars in the philosophy of mind and researchers in cognitive science hold that

---

[7] See commentaries by Barrouillet and Markovits (pp. 330–1) claiming that the SOC does not account well for human deductive reasoning; Bornstein (pp. 332–3), who holds that subliminal (unconscious) presentations yielding stronger affect-based effects than supraliminal presentations cannot be explained with the SOC model; Jimenez (p. 342), stating that the SOC does not provide a satisfactory account for learning processes and their products; Keisler and Willingham (pp. 342–3), who claim that complex motor skills cannot be explained adequately with the SOC; Lambert (pp. 344–5), finding that a number of phenomena, for example, unconscious semantic processing and various neuropsychological syndromes including prosopagnosia, neglect, split brain syndrome, and some types of amnesia cannot be sufficiently explained with conscious representations alone; and Parisse and Cohen (pp. 349–50), Rivera-Gaxiola and Silva-Pereyra (pp. 352–3), and Yamauchi (p. 360), all of whom find the SOC model not satisfactory to account for different aspects of language acquisition and use.

"Mental life is posited as co-extensive with consciousness" (p. 299). Recognizing that this definitional fiat is not much of an argument, Perruchet and Vinter are not willing to leave the matter there. This is to their credit, but their next step is no less problematic. They contend that since

> [1] the mentalistic view rejects notions of unconscious rule abstraction, computation, analysis, reasoning, and inference ... [and, 2] unconscious representations have no other function than to enter into these activities, [therefore, 3] eliminating the possibility of these activities actually makes the overall notion of unconscious representation objectless. (p. 299)

Essentially, this three-step argument is supposed to demonstrate that unconscious representations have no functional role. But all three parts of the argument are flawed. Part 1 is really no more than a version of the definitional fiat above—*unconscious* rule abstraction, computation, analysis, reasoning, and inference are rejected because these processes are mental and mental processes must be conscious. And parts two and three of the argument not only take the first part as true, but further assert, without argument, just what they are trying to further prove—namely that given no unconscious rule abstraction, computation, and so on there can be no other[8] functional role for unconscious representations. Therefore, on any or all of these grounds, the argument for unconscious representations having no functional role does not hold.

Second, there is a threat of vicious circularity in the claim of isomorphism between conscious representations and the world. Perruchet and Vinter hold that since there are no unconscious processes operating on unconscious representations, the main question they must address is, How can one "account for the fact that the content of phenomenal experience is, even in a limited sense, isomorphic to the world?" (p. 302). This question seems either incoherent or circular. For on Perruchet and Vinter's account, how can there fail to be isomorphism? Given that for them the structure of the *known* world consists of the total collections of conscious representations of the world (and the usual extensions via technical tools), and given that our phenomenal experience likewise consists of just these conscious representations, how could they *not* match?

The question of the relations between what obtains in the world and what we, through our representations of any sort can know of the world are fiendishly difficult (and very interesting). In no way do I hold that merely reintroducing unconscious representations would provide satisfying explanations. What I do

---

[8] The use of the word "other" here shows that Perruchet and Vinter tacitly grant that if unconscious rule abstraction, computation, reasoning, and inference were to exist, then they would have to admit that unconscious representations do have a functional role.

hold, however, is that a mentalistic theory that included unconscious representations would not have to claim general isomorphism between representations and the world in the first place. The questionable status of this claim of isomorphism is the next problematic matter.

Third, why do representations and what they represent need to be isomorphic for representations to do the work of representing in the first place? Certainly this is not a necessary condition for ordinary conscious representations. Take two obvious examples: both musical notations and words represent by convention, not isomorphism. The physical item named and denoted by the word "pencil" is in no way isomorphic to the word "p-e-n-c-i-l" which represents it.

But consider the authors' own comments on the case of a picture of a pencil on a slide in a slide projector:

> Everybody would agree that the picture fulfills its representative function for a human perceiver when it is projected on a screen. But what about this picture when it is not displayed? It is only a pattern of colored pixels on a film … The storage format does not matter, because a stored picture has no other function than making possible the subsequent generations of the picture. What is kept over time is the possibility of generating the picture again through appropriate procedures … which are not [themselves] embedded in the stored picture. (p. 328, note 1 referring to p. 299)

Clearly, Perruchet and Vinter are implying that the pattern of colored pixels on film is not a representation.

But what if one could understand a representation to be that which has been abstracted from something meaningful such that the same meaningful something can be reliably reconstructed? Wouldn't this non-isomorphic stored version *be* a representation—much as a specific set of musical notations represent a specific piece of music? Perruchet and Vinter would have to say "no" owing to the isomorphism requirement. But, they do not *argue* for necessary isomorphism; they merely impose it as a necessary feature for any representations at all and therefore for unconscious representations. They state that "the possibility of generating the conscious representation of past experience does not mean in any way that this representation has enduring existence as such (i.e. serves its function) in a putative unconscious system" (p. 328, note 1 referring to p. 299). The phrase "enduring existence *as such*" implies "enduring existence *in the same form*." Here Perruchet and Vinter try to make a case against these analogs to unconscious representations insofar as they are not isomorphic to conscious representations—but it is Perruchet and Vinter who imposed this condition of isomorphism in the first place! Thus, with the faulty premise that Perruchet and Vinter originated to the effect that unconscious representations must be isomorphic to conscious representations to represent and thereby play the functional role representations play, Perruchet and Vinter argue against any unconscious representations at all.

The *fourth* matter revisits the presumption of isomorphism, the question of functional role, and the problem of definitional fiat. Perruchet and Vinter allow that associative processes are unconscious. But seemingly for no reason other than that these processes do operate unconsciously, Perruchet and Vinter do not consider them to be mental processes (pp. 299–300). This is the obverse of the definitional argument that the truly mental processes of rule abstraction, computation, analysis, reasoning, and inference must be conscious and cannot be unconscious because they are mental. Of further interest, Perruchet and Vinter's apparent by-definition claim that unconscious associative processes are not mental is quite reminiscent of Searle's conclusions that the associative/transformative processes cannot be mental.

But if we were to consider unconscious associative processes to be truly mental, would we actually get an absurd result? Suppose we stipulate that these unconscious associative processes (1) do not perform the higher level rational mental operations such as rule abstraction, computation, analysis, reasoning, and inference; but that instead (2) they do carry on the primary process type operations of transforming—processes such as the displacements and conden-sations evident in dreams and psychological pathological symptoms, as well as in slips of the tongue, parapraxes, daydreams, and certain types of categoriza-tions. Is there something absurd in allowing these associative/transformative processes as *mental* activity? I think not. What if we then took a further step, allowing the possibility that these unconscious associative mental processes could operate on non-isomorphic precursors to conscious representations? Then these non-isomorphic precursors to conscious representations, better known by their usual name of *unconscious representations*, would have a func-tional role as the objects of these unconscious associative mental processes. Far from having an absurd result, we would have a theory of mind more parsi-monious than Perruchet and Vinter's SOC, a theory requiring fewer circular presumptions and by-definition declarations.

The nature of psychoanalytic theory: Lessons from geometry and space[9]

Having addressed skeptical theorists who would have a theory of mind with neither unconscious representations nor mental associative processes, the task for the remainder of the chapter is more positive (in the sense of having to

---

[9] Much of what follows in this section is taken from Brakel (1994a). This is an article, "Lessons from the Geometry of Space" and it appears in the *International Journal of Psychoanalysis*. Vol. 75: 39–49.

provide something rather than refute something) and more difficult. Let me begin by returning to the title of this chapter: "Just what sort of theory is psychoanalytic theory?" To answer this question it is necessary to investigate two further questions. First, how can we know (in another or in ourselves) the unconscious, when it is by definition not available to consciousness? Second, beyond even the possibility of knowing the unconscious, how can we know not only its contents, but also the very laws posited to govern unconscious operations—the primary processes? In *The Unconscious* Freud (1915b) raises the three central issues I will examine here regarding knowing the unconscious and its nature: He states, (1) "Our right to assume the existence of something mental that is unconscious and to employ that assumption for the purpose of scientific work is disputed in many quarters. To this we reply that our assumption of the unconscious is *necessary and legitimate*" (p. 166). He then asks and answers, (2) "How are we to arrive at a knowledge of the unconscious? It is of course only as something conscious that we know it, after it has undergone transformation or translation into something conscious" (p. 166). Freud then asserts, (3) "we have to take into account the fact that analytic investigation reveals some of these latent [unconscious] processes as having characteristics and peculiarities which seem alien to us, or even incredible, and which run directly counter to the attributes of consciousness with which we are familiar" (p. 170).

Indeed, like Freud, I hold that positing the unconscious is an assumption necessary for psychoanalytic theory and method. However, his claim for legitimacy is premature. As is true for any postulate posited to account for observations and thereafter assumed, the assumption itself can be proved neither by the observational data nor by the data generated by the method. Instead, evidential warrant must be sought outside the method (Grunbaum 1984). This is the case no matter how well the assumption brings coherence and consistency to a theory, its method and findings; as is obviously true with the assumption of a dynamic, psychologically meaningful unconscious and psychoanalysis. Thus as a compliment to research on psychoanalysis using non-psychoanalytic methods,[10] I now will investigate arguments for positing

---

[10] A great deal of research has been carried out in this manner at the Hunt Memorial Laboratory for Unconscious Processes headed by Howard Shevrin and codirected by the author and Michael Snodgrass. This research team has also made use of convergent psychoanalytic and non-psychoanalytic methods. For example, Shevrin *et al.* (1992), and Shevrin *et al.*(1996), used the psychoanalytic clinical method in conjunction with two methods, neither of which presumes the dynamic unconscious—the subliminal method and the evoked-response potential method—to provide convergent evidence for unconscious processes and unconscious conflict.

the unconscious and knowing its nature, not from within any psychoanalytic framework, but by analogy to a similar set of problems in the realm of geometry and space—problems considered by philosophers of science to have been already reasonably well worked out.

One of the advantages, which I hope further justifies my use of geometry and space as a model for epistemological and ontological considerations about the unconscious, involves the standing of Euclidean geometry of ordinary-dimension space as the spatial organizer, functioning along with forward moving time and some modern version of Kant's 12 necessary categories of thought, as that which is necessary for constituting human thought and thereby making human understanding possible. I will propose, starting from Freud's assertion that we can know the unconscious only via its conscious derivatives, that conscious mentation, particularly the secondary processes that predominate, conform not only to everyday logical thought, but also to the Kantian categories (along with forward moving time and Euclidean space). The unconscious and primary processes, like non-Euclidean subatomic particle space and astronomical macro-space, in contrast, are outside the Kantian categories. My claim is that by using these better understood, but similarly "outside-the-categories" phenomena to construct an analogy, we can begin to account for the "peculiarities which seem alien ... even incredible," of the latent unconscious primary processes to which Freud referred.

Kantian categories and primary and secondary processes

In *The Unconscious*, Freud (1915b) set out some of the characteristics of what he then called the system "Unconscious and its primary process." (1) "There are in this system no negation, no doubt, no degrees of certainty" (p. 186), (2) "The processes of the system *Ucs.* are *timeless*; i.e. they are not ordered temporally, are not altered by the passage of time" (p. 187), (3) "The *Ucs.* processes pay just as little regard to *reality*. They are subject to the pleasure principle" (p. 187), (4) The instinctual drives, wishes, and ideas comprising this system strive for discharge; they are exempt from mutual contradiction, and can achieve discharge via displacement (one entity standing for another) and condensation (one entity standing for many) (pp. 186–7). In addition to displacement and condensation, other associational/nonlogical operations are considered to be part of the primary processes. Thus, part for whole representations and associations by contiguity in time and/or space take the place of ordinary "logical" connections, whereas the operations we routinely (and consciously) use for commonsense as well as scientific understanding are largely part of the secondary processes. Following Freud (1915, pp. 186–8) the secondary processes are marked by reality-testing, delay of discharge, and restricted use of condensation and displacement. Moreover for the secondary processes principles of standard logic obtain, identity is singular and within ordinary time and space constraints, causality is assumed, and crossing frames of reference for categorizations and sometimes even for associations is largely unacceptable.

It has occurred to me (Brakel 1984, 1994a; and see Chapter 4) that Freud's secondary process operating principles seem to be modernized versions of Kant's "categories of thought necessary for understanding."[11] Indeed, the same "something non-trivial about the nature of the world" (Sklar 1974, p. 83) results from both Kant's (1781/1787) assertion that to obtain coherent experience of our world we order the world according to Euclidean space, forward moving time, and the 12 categories, and our recognition that as adults we cannot help but automatically utilize secondary process capacities. The "something non-trivial" added in both cases is, of course, knowledge about the nature of human understanding itself. But note that nothing has been gained regarding knowledge of the world independent of how we organize it in order to experience it; and no knowledge has been gained about the psychological unconscious and its laws and contents. Even the ontological status of these entities remains in question, as the world independent of our understanding and the unconscious remain outside of the categories.

Models

Were it not for the concept of models, the plan for this chapter—to learn more about the unconscious and its nature by analogy, would fail. As it is, three different applications of models contribute. Most simply, the epistemologic/ontologic problems of geometry and space are being used as a model for analogous problems regarding the unconscious and its operating principles. The other two uses of models are intertwined: models can generate outside-the-categories possibilities (outside-the-Kantian categories/outside-the-secondary processes); and models can allow possibilities outside-the-categories to be

---

[11] Here is Kant's (1781/1787 [1965], p. 113) table of categories. He arranges them into four groups, each with three categories. I—*Of Quantity*: Unity, Plurality, Totality; II—*Of Quality*: Reality, Negation, Limitation; III—*Of Relation*: Of Inherence and Subsistence, Of Causality and Dependence (cause and effect), Of Community (reciprocity between agent and patient); IV—*Of Modality*: Possibility–Impossibility, Existence–Nonexistence, Necessity–Contingency.

assimilated to the categories and thereby coherently apprehended. What follows demonstrates these last two applications of models in the geometry of space case.

Various mathematicians and philosophers of science have stated rather emphatically that Kant was wrong to consider Euclidean space a necessary *a priori* component in the way the human mind organizes experience in order to have experience. Even in textbooks of the geometries it is stated as a fact that "Gauss' discovery of non-Euclidean geometry refuted Kant's position that Euclidean space is *inherent in the structure of our mind*" (Greenberg 1972, p. 145). But did Gauss (and colleagues) really *discover* a non-Euclidean geometry? My own view is that they did not. Rather, they constructed or derived such from the Euclidean, after making an assumption different from Euclid's axiom of parallels. Reichenbach (1951) attacked Kant's views forcefully too:

> The principles which Kant had considered to be indispensable ... have been recognized as holding only to a limited degree. Important laws of classical physics were found to apply only to phenomena occurring in our ordinary environment. For astronomical and for sub-microscopic dimensions they had to be replaced by laws of the new physics and this fact alone makes it obvious that they were empirical laws and not laws forced on us by reason itself. (p. 125)

But Reichenbach (1958) went on to describe the mathematician's procedure of "'visualizing' non-Euclidean geometry by means of Euclidean geometry... based upon the mathematical fact that non-Euclidean geometry can be mapped upon Euclidean space" (p. 49). Thus Euclidean geometry provides the model (1) that with certain transformations produces the new outside-the-categories non-Euclidean geometry, and (2) provides that which the outside-the-category geometry is mapped onto, not only validating this new geometry mathematically, but also enabling it to be visualized and understood by what seems even more clearly to be our native and necessary Euclidean understanding.

Before examining matters of interest—the epistemologic/ontologic problems of the unconscious and its operating laws—I must briefly review four different solutions to analogous problems in the better accepted theory to be used as the model, that concerning the geometry of space. The problem, simply stated, is what geometry best describes space—Euclidean geometry or one of the non-Euclidean geometries?

Poincare and the geometric conventionalist view of space

Poincare (1907) demonstrated that non-Euclidean geometry is as consistent as Euclidean geometry. In fact, the non-Euclidean geometries, based on and understood in terms of various Euclidean models (i.e. models based on different segments of Euclidean three-space), must be consistent if Euclidean geometry is consistent. But consistency does not imply truth. How can truth be ascertained? Conventionalists claim that since all possible observational data will always lead as readily to a Euclidean understanding of space as to a non-Euclidean, and since these are incompatible, "two alternative total theories" (Sklar 1974, p. 117), one cannot on the basis of any observational evidence make a determination between them. Poincare nonetheless advocated that a choice be made, but a choice *by convention*. Finding Euclidean geometry "simpler," Poincare favored Euclidean geometry. But this raises the question: simpler in what sense? The question suggests that there are other positions to be considered. (See my criticism of Perruchet and Vinter's "parsimonious" theory of the mental above, pp. 20–24.)

The a *priori*-ist position

The a *priori*-ist position under discussion here is not the same as Kant's view that it is an *a priori* and necessary matter that Euclidean space grounds any human understanding of space. On the contrary for this group, the question of the geometry of space is not beyond possible refutation by empirical experience, and experimentation and observation play a critical role (Sklar 1974, p. 129). But regarding the problem at hand, it is claimed that the two incompatible theories are *to this point* each equally well able to describe all the available experimental data. The a *priori*-ist then turns to the structural features of the theories themselves, evaluating their relative initial plausibility, simplicity, generality, and explanatory power in the face of experimental and observational findings (Sklar 1974, p. 131). The a *priori*-ist is thus an a *priori*-ist not about any particular theory but concerning the structure and methodological principles of theory itself. Perruchet and Vinter would be properly classified as a *priori*-ists in that they hold that their theory of mind suffices while it is simpler theoretically than any theory of mind including unconscious representations. Note that my argument against Perruchet and Vinter was not against their *priori*-ist stance, but rather was a refutation of the claim that their theory of mind was theoretically simpler.

Reichenbach's reductionism

For Reichenbach (and Eddington, the physicist) the two theories of geometry are only apparently mutually exclusive. In fact, they claim that whenever a situation exists where no data can *ever* provide grounds for a decision between two alternatives, the two alternatives are actually different expressions or translations of the same theory. An account challenging to both the conventionalist and a *priori*-ist positions, for Reichenbach the view that non-Euclidean and

Euclidean geometry are two expressions of one theory of space implies that one version can be "simpler" than the other. But he cautioned that one must differentiate between inductive simplicity and mere "descriptive simplicity which has nothing to do with truth" (Reichenbach 1958, p. 35). Reichenbach argues for the inductive simplicity of non-Euclidean geometry:

> From his [Einstein's] general theory of relativity he derived the conclusion that in astronomic dimensions the nature of space is non-Euclidean. This does not contradict Gauss' measurements according to which the geometry of terrestrial dimensions is Euclidean, because it is a general property of non-Euclidean geometry that for [relatively] small areas it is practically identical with the Euclidean geometry. (1951, p. 130)

But there is still the matter of Kant's claim that we necessarily organize experience in an Euclidean manner. Indeed Reichenbach does acknowledge our continued need for Euclidean models, attributes this to "habit" (1958, p. 48), and likens the capacity to use non-Euclidean theory to that of learning a foreign (nonnative) language. But shouldn't his reductionist position have to accommodate the observation that human geometrical eyes universally employ natively and naturally the inductively more complex Euclidean geometry?

Reductionism in two directions: Epistemologic and ontologic considerations

Embedded in the geometry of space dilemma are two issues—an ontologic question about the nature of the cosmos and an epistemologic one concerning how the cosmos can be known. Can any of the above positions deal with both successfully? Let us return to models in both their generative and conservative roles. A model generates outside-the-category possibilities that are not yet coherent—non-Euclidean geometries modeled on, but different from Euclidean geometry can be posited. A model can also subsume the outside-the-category material—the non-Euclidean geometries can be mapped onto the Euclidean model. In both cases certain *transformations* are required: (1) to derive non-Euclidean geometry from Euclidean geometry epistemologically, and (2) to map non-Euclidean geometry, the more ontologically fundamental theory of space, back onto the Euclidean theory. I am using the term *transformation* in favor of Reichenbach's term *translation* to suggest that, transformations involve learning something "non-trivial" about the world. Transformations, as I am proposing them, are themselves outside of the categories, but not unknowable entities, in the very modest sense that the use of a particular set of transformations, compared with others possible, provides us with genuine, new, nontrivial knowledge. (See p. 34 below.)

But if transformations do carry nontrivial information and if transformations are required to travel each leg of an epistemological round trip, first by deriving non-Euclidean geometries *from* Euclidean geometry and then by mapping the new geometries *back onto* the Euclidean model, any explanatory theory must accommodate what is clearly the relative simplicity of Euclidean geometry *epistemologically*, as well as the relative simplicity *ontologically* of non-Euclidean geometric theories of space. Of all the candidates, it seems that Reichenbach's reductionism can work, but only with an important modi-fication. It must be employed in two different directions: ontologically the non-Euclidean theories are inductively simpler; but epistemologically, Euclidean geometry clearly is the simpler theory—and this is not merely "descriptive simplicity which has nothing to do with truth"—it is simplicity that has to do with epistemic truth.

Lessons applied: On knowing the unconscious and its nature

Although the ontological and epistemological problems of the unconscious and primary process mentation can be seen as analogous to those of space and non-Euclidean geometry, there are a few important differences. Unconscious mentation with primary process organization on the one hand, and ordinary, conscious, mature, secondary process (Kantian category) thinking on the other, are not two alternative, incompatible whole psychological theories of mind, each equally conforming to the same body of observational data. Nor can they be seen as two versions or translations expressing a single theory of mind. Instead, most analysts hold that there is a dual operation of both sorts of mentation in every psychological event, such that causal explanations can be provided even for those psychological events (such as symptoms and parap-raxes) that seem from a secondary process framework incoherent, once uncon-scious aspects of mentation (often in a primary process mode) can be assumed and understood.

  Despite these differences, however, several features of the above analysis of the geometry of space dilemma do seem applicable to that of the unconscious and its nature. Thus what follows is a presentation of four views in which the lessons of geometry and space are applied to the unconscious and primary process.

Kantian skepticism

Once we have reached cognitive maturity, humans necessarily utilize the secondary processes/Kantian categories to organize experience coherently. It is a puzzle then as to what can be said about unconscious mentation and a mode of operations (the primary process) different from the categories. The Kantian skeptic would hold that the existence of unconscious mentation cannot be ruled out nor can it be established; likewise with respect to attributions regarding the nature of the unconscious. What can be *known* is only this: constitutive of a coherent experience is that it be organized by our necessary secondary process categories for understanding. Indeed Freud's most momentous achievement involved a most creative turn on just this fact. By taking symptoms and other behaviors that had been regarded as random biological residues, senseless in themselves, and positing that they had unconscious causes operating according to the primary processes, Freud found that these bizarre behaviors became coherent, meaningful, and capable of admitting of the standard Kantian category/secondary process application. However, precisely because for Freud this newfound coherence was totally dependent upon *positing* unconscious psychological causes organized in a primary process fashion, this move cannot be used to overcome the skepticism of the Kantian skeptic, a skepticism about exactly what Freud posited and then took for granted.

The psychological conventionalist position

As the geometrical conventionalist chooses one or another geometry, but only by convention, the dilemma of unconscious mentation and primary process provides an analogous choice to psychological theorists: whether or not to posit omnipresent and significantly meaningful unconscious mentation (and its characteristic form of operation). For the psychological conventionalist, as for his/her geometrical counterpart, no amount or type of observational data can ever provide an evidential basis for or against this posit. But a choice must be made and so it is by convention. Theorists whose arguments against unconscious mentation are founded on definitional matters—for example, the mental is by definition conscious and rational—belong in this conventionalist group.

The psychological *a priori*-ists

As with the geometry of space problem, *a priori*-ists with respect to the unconscious mentation dilemma use considerations pertaining to the theories themselves to decide between two total theories—one positing a dynamic unconscious with primary process mentation, and the other not. Evidence is useful for the *a priori*-ist, but the premise is that currently available evidence is not sufficient to make the determination. Thus inspecting each theory for its simplicity, generality of its domain, and explanatory power of the phenomena under study, the decision is made. As was discussed above, Perruchet and Vinter (2002) claimed that the simpler theory was the one without unconscious representations and argued that the phenomena of interest could still be satisfactorily explained. I argued that the theory of mind without unconscious representation might be "descriptively" simpler (to now adopt Reichenbach's terms), but structurally was not simpler. Other commentators felt that Perruchet and Vinter's account was either not able to account for an adequately wide range of phenomena (not sufficiently general) or not able to explain some phenomena of interest satisfactorily (not having sufficient explanatory power). (For references to these commentaries see footnote 6, this chapter.)

By the same criteria used by Perruchet and Vinter—simplicity, generalizability, and explanatory power—most psychoanalytic theorists come to the opposite conclusion, namely that the theory of mind including unconscious and primary process mentation should be favored. However, even if this stands (and I have argued for this above), the psychoanalysts have another problem: they overextend the *a priori*-ist claim believing that their theory, owing to its simplicity, generalizability, and explanatory power, has also some standing with respect to evidential warrant. And this is just not true. Evidential warrant for unconscious and primary process mentation cannot be gained even if it is the case that a theory of mind which includes them is structurally simpler; and despite the fact that any analyst can amass scores of examples in which assuming unconscious and primary process mentation convincingly explains a tremendous variety of otherwise seemingly incomprehensible psychological events. Warrant for the existence of unconscious mentation and its primary process nature simply cannot be established in this fashion.

This is as far as the question of knowing the unconscious—knowing its existence and that of its primary process modes of operation—usually goes. But perhaps for the fourth and final view we can push things a little further by investigating a bidirectional ontologic and epistemologic reductionism, one modeled on the bidirectional reductionism applied to the geometry of space problem. It follows in two parts.

Epistemological reductionism

Remembering that, for Reichenbach and the geometry of space reductionists, the Euclidean and non-Euclidean theories of space were really one theory in different translations, let us reconsider to what extent the two theories of the mind—the unconscious primary process mentation and the Kantian category type secondary processes—could be considered two versions of just one theory. We can legitimately claim that we can only understand (know) that which we deem unconscious and primary process according to the conscious, secondary process/Kantian categories we necessarily apply for all experience (see also Chapter 4). Thus, a dream replete with primary process content reflective of unconscious processes becomes comprehensible only in Kantian category/secondary process terms. A patient reports that "The dream was 'funny'. Dr X didn't look like Dr X, but somehow she was. At the same time she both was and became Mr O. Next, a glass fell hard on a concrete floor, but it didn't break." Note that the Kantian categories are applied and the dream material fitted in, but only in the negative, with negativity itself being a Kantian category/secondary process operation.

But granted that Kantian categories/secondary process are applied so that primary process material is now organized in a secondary process model, can we learn something about the primary processes if we can understand *how* the secondary process model is made, what transformations are required? Again I am making a distinction between translations and transformations, claiming the latter carry nontrivial information.[12] As such the various different sorts of transformations necessary to bring primary process material into a secondary process model can be recognized, observed, studied, and compared to gain nontrivial knowledge. So, for example, in the dream material just above, the secondary processes subsume the primary process elements only after the primary process material is transformed. The dream content itself is *indifferent* to singular identity (She was Dr X and Mr O), forward moving time (Dr X both was and was becoming Mr O), and cause and effect (the glass fell and did not break); but it is transformed to content that *violates* singular identity, forward moving time, and causality. In this way (and it seems paradoxical), by being content that is organized as *not* causal, *not* following forward moving time, and *not* behaving according to singular identity, the primary process dream content is transformed, by the transformational operator of negation, to content that *is* actually organized according to the secondary process (Kantian) categories. The primary process version alone, without negations applied to the secondary process/Kantian category model could not be understood.

By adopting this sort of epistemologic reductionism, whereby unconscious and primary process mentation, in order to be known must be subsumed by secondary process/Kantian category models via transformations, we have gained some nontrivial knowledge of unconscious and primary process mentation. What about the ontological considerations?

---

12 To quickly demonstrate the level of difference between translation and transformation, consider the following (admittedly loose) analogy. If the changes needed to dye a green velvet skirt purple stand for a translation, changing a green velvet skirt to green velvet pants—entailing additions, subtractions, and recombinations—would be illustrative of a transformation.

Attempting an ontological reductionism

Just above, we have seen a type of reductionism whereby all primary process mentation can be understood *epistemologically*, but only via transformations to secondary process models. This parallels a similar reductionism in that the understanding of non-Euclidean geometries of space goes through epistemologically via the Euclidean geometry of space. Is there also the possibility of an analogue to the spatial/physical reductionism—the *ontological* reductionism in which the geometry of the cosmos can be singularly non-Euclidean, while ordinary-sized areas seem Euclidean, because (as Reichenbach, [1951], p. 138 puts it) at these dimensions the two geometries are "practically identical"? I suggest that we can employ what I will call a developmental/ontological reductionism; and that as in the geometry of space case it goes in the opposite direction from the epistemologic reduction.

The developmental/ontologic reduction is predicated on what are taken as the basic facts about unconscious and primary process mentation vs. conscious and secondary process mentation. Namely that the unconscious and primary processes are primary and ubiquitous, developing very early on and remaining as a background even in the most conscious and rational psychological events; while the later developing conscious/secondary process/Kantian category type of mentation, is more highly organized, and like everyday-sized space, can be applied to only a relatively small subset of psychological events.[13] So, for example, one can readily observe the predominance of primary process mentation in much of the thinking activity of pre-school age children, in dreams, daydreams, delusions, hallucinations, and all manner of psychological pathological symptoms. Less obvious, psychoanalysts nonetheless maintain that even the most rational, highest level, alert conscious wakeful thoughts develop from, and are partly composed of, ever-present unconscious and primary process goings-on. Freud, in his last systematic writing says as much with no equivocation: "No; being conscious cannot be the essence of what is psychical. It is only a quality of what is psychical, and an inconsistent quality at that—one that is far oftener absent than present. The psychical, whatever its nature may be, is in itself [largely] unconscious" (1940, p. 383).

---

[13] Now there is an important difference: Everyday-sized space can be properly described by either Euclidean or non-Euclidean theories, while primary process principles alone will not suffice for a description of a rational thought or action. This owes to the fact that secondary process thought is not a special manifestation of primary process thought, applicable in just certain selected psychological events.

Conclusions from geometry lessons

I have suggested that there is a deep analogy between the epistemologic and ontologic problems of the geometry of space and those in the general psychological theory of mind. The geometry of space problems involve Euclidean vs. non-Euclidean theories; the psychological theory of mind problems involve theories which include unconscious and primary process mentation vs. those that do not. Using the better-studied geometry of space problem as a model, I have proposed (1) an epistemological reductionism in which the unconscious and primary process can only be known through conscious and secondary processes, much as epistemologically non-Euclidean geometries are dependent on Euclidean geometries, and (2) an ontologic reductionism in the opposite direction, in which the unconscious and primary process are foundational and ubiquitous, while the conscious and secondary process mentation exist in only a small subset of psychological events. This reductionism is similar to (albeit not identical with) the geometry of space situation, in which the non-Euclidean geometries can account for space of any size, whereas both Euclidean and non-Euclidean can work for ordinary-sized space.

If this argument by analogy is successful and I have been able to show that there can be some legitimacy in both knowing that which is unconscious and knowing about its primary process nature, no psychoanalyst will be surprised; that is, what he/she has presumed all along. But that is one of the points of this chapter. Methodologically, assumptions cannot be strengthened from within a method or theory that assumes them. Hence the geometry lesson is intended as a set of speculative arguments, outside psychoanalytic theory, through which credence can be gained via argument by analogy to the better-studied problems of the geometry of space, for basic fundaments of psychoanalytic theory—namely, that there exists an unconscious and that, though by definition it is a realm of which we cannot be directly aware, we can nonetheless gain nontrivial knowledge of its nature, contents, and processes.

Chapter conclusions

The general psychoanalytic theory of mind presents two immediate problems to philosophers and cognitive scientists: it posits a dynamic meaningful representational unconscious and an unconscious with organizing principles different from those organizing much of ordinary adult conscious wakeful thought. After first addressing skeptics who argue against the very notion of unconscious representations (Searle) and those who argue against the need for them (Perruchet and Vinter), the work of this chapter centers on distinguishing between epistemologic and ontologic aspects of the two immediate problems.

It is demonstrated that some ground can be gained in both domains by investigating an analogous set of problems in the area of the geometry of space.

On the way to this conclusion several claims were made, among them that, (1) the epistemological problems for the psychoanalytic theory of mind are essentially problems in Kantian epistemology and (2) that Freud's secondary process mentation can be shown to map quite well onto Kant's categories necessary for understanding. In Part II both of these claims will be explored in much more detail.

Part II

Epistemological issues

Part II, consisting of Chapters 3 and 4, is more directly concerned with issues of epistemology, specifically investigating Freudian primary and secondary process in Kantian terms. Chapter 3 examines a little heralded precursor to Freud's primary process in Kant's ontology of thinking. Chapter 4 investigates the Kantian epistemological dilemma in knowing primary process mentation.

Chapter 3

Did Kant precede Freud on a-rational thought?

'Unusual' human experiences: Kant, Freud, and an associationist principle[1]

Kant famously held that there are 12 categories of understanding necessary *a priori* to ground human experience,[2] where human experience can be taken to include the perception of objects "objectively" and the ordinary rational cognition of mature adults. There are however other "unusual" human experiences, most notably dream and hallucinatory states, and much of the thinking of the very young, all of which seem to be grounded by some other organizing principle, prior to the Kantian categories. I want to make the case that this principle is an associationist one, organized by contiguity in time and/or space; and further that such an associationist principle is prior to and necessary for Kant's categories to operate.[3] Since Kant himself held this, although not so

---

[1] This section is a revised version of an article that first appeared in Brakel (2003). "Unusual" human experiences: Kant, Freud, and an associationist law. *Theoria et Historica Scientificarum*: Special issue on Unconscious Perception and Communication: Evolutionary, Cognitive and Psychoanalytic Perspectives. Vol. 7: 109–16.

[2] Kant's (1781/1787 [1965] A80/B106, p. 113) table of categories is listed in Chapter 2, footnote 11. Note that in this chapter in addition to page references for Kant's *Critique of Pure Reason*, there will be either an A or a B followed by a number denoting the passage. A refers to the first (1781) edition and B to the second (1787) edition.

[3] The search for a grounding organizing principle for basic experiences like the constituting of objects as objects has for centuries involved debates between *empiricistism* vs. *nativism*. In these debates the empiricists held that a passive registration of associated sensations added up to final objects, while the nativists contended that an active mind constructed them on the basis of inborn templates. A version of this—associationism vs. Gestalt psychology—was important even in mid-twentieth century psychology. For example, Gardner Murphy in the respected 1933 textbook *General Psychology* states that "Perception is either the association of sensory particles with one another, or it is the unified act of the mind, by which the separate parts are reacted to and somehow made into one" (p. 629). He goes on (p. 631) to describe the program of the Gestalt psychologists (namely Koffka

famously,[4] the purpose of this chapter is not to refute Kant. Rather it is to demonstrate that experiences so organized by the associationist law and those organized by the categories map very well onto the different sorts of experiences mediated by two types of mentation posited by Freud—the "primary processes" and the "secondary processes," respectively. Discovering this mapping can help psychoanalytic theory by providing some convergent support for its posits; and it can make vivid a lesser known piece of Kantian philosophy of mind as it is demonstrated in everyday clinical psychoanalytic observations.

Introduction

Kant in the *Critique of Pure Reason* (1781, 1787) argues that the categories for understanding are necessary *a priori* for knowledge of objects, really for any understanding at all. He further argues that even though these principles of our cognitive functioning (the *a priori* categories) are not knowable empirically, we can have "transcendental" knowledge of them. The *a priori* part of his claim means that since these categories are needed to *even* have any experience, they must be prior to any experience. But what does he mean by "transcendental knowledge"? He wrote, "I entitle *transcendental* all knowledge which is occupied not so much with objects as with the mode of our knowledge of objects, in so far as this mode of knowledge is to be possible a priori" (A11–12/B25, p. 59). And he continued: "[transcendental] proof proceeds by showing that experience itself, and therefore the object of experience, would be impossible without a connection of this kind" (A783/B811, p. 621). Patricia Kitcher (1990) summarizes: "transcendental knowledge concerns how we know objects…. Transcendental knowledge is established by transcendental proofs,

---

1925; Kohler 1929), who call for the study of what Murphy terms "the lumps of experience," that is, the unitary, global totals, as innately given templates by which the mind is active and can organize even shifting parts.

However, to frame this debate in either/or terms has always been highly problematic. As Kitcher (1990, p. 80) exclaims, "the obvious answer is 'both'. To understand how we are able to construct representations of objects, for example, we need to look at both the patterns of our sensory stimulations and the way the mind uses those patterns to construct representations." In this spirit, I want to make clear that the associationist principle discussed in this chapter—that very principle rejected by Kant as the organizing synthetic principle for grounding experience—is a principle of mind predicated not on mere passive registration of sensations, but on the active organization of the massive numbers of incoming sensations, albeit in an associative way, and not (yet) according to the categories.

[4] I thank Ian Proops who pointed this out to me (Personal Communication 2002).

which show that experience would be impossible but for the *a priori* origins of certain features of our cognition" (p. 15).

Kant famously argues that the 12 categories of understanding are the features of our cognition that provide the principles transcendentally necessary *a priori* for combining and transforming the countless inputs to our multimodal sensory systems into any conscious understanding, any knowledge of objects, and even any conscious experience at all. According to Kant, "All synthesis … even that which renders perception possible, is subject to the categories; and since experience is knowledge by means of connected perceptions, the categories are conditions of the possibility of experience" (B161, p. 171). Associationism is another possible combinatory principle—but it is one that Kant argued could not ground human experience.

In this chapter I will make a case for an associationist law that is necessary anterior (i.e. prior) to the categories. To state it differently, I want to claim that the transcendentally necessary categories are themselves in an important sense dependent upon earlier association-based organizations. Interestingly, as I will discuss below, Kant himself would have little disagreement with this. Instead, a point of contention concerns Kant's use of the term "human experience." For Kant, only *category*-based mentation, yielding knowledge and perception of objects-as-we-know-them, constitutes human experience. While a case can be made that some sorts of human experiences are based on associationist organization—for example dream experiences, hallucinations, and the thinking of very young children—it is clear that Kant meant normal, everyday rational, mature human experience. In my view, arguing this merely rhetorical point would be of little interest. On the other hand it *is* important to highlight the necessity of an associationist law upon which the categories depend because this will allow a Freudian posit central to psychoanalysis—that there are two very differently organized types of mental processes, the "primary processes" and the "secondary processes"—to be grounded in Kantian philosophy of mind.

The primary and secondary processes

Reviewing the psychoanalytic posit of the primary processes (corollary one), by 1900, Freud (*The Interpretation of Dreams* Vol. 4 & 5) had clearly delineated two types of mentation. He termed our more familiar everyday rational sort of thinking "secondary process" mentation. Secondary processes consist of mechanisms, states, and contents that constitute much of what we experience consciously as our ordinary rationality. Kant's categories for understanding can be seen to comprise the necessary organizing principles for secondary process rational thinking (see Brakel 1984, 1994a) insofar as the secondary processes are tensed (i.e. they are about events in specific real time: past, present, or future), reality tested, and admit of no contradictions. Freud's "primary processes" on the other hand, although still mental and contentful, lack one or more of these hallmarks of the rational. They are tenseless; they involve no conception of the past or future—they are always about an "unexamined present." With primary process mentation there is no reality testing—no considerations of truth and falsity, in other words distinctions cannot be made among what *is*, what *may be possible*, and what *cannot be*. Finally, the primary processes tolerate contradictions. (This can be seen most readily with young children, for example, a child given the choice of going in the car with Mommy or staying home with Daddy sometimes wants to do both.)[5] Clearly, synthesis according to the Kantian categories does not occur with this sort of mentation. Consequently, something quite different from our usual conscious experience, and even different from our usual knowledge of objects as determinate objects, results from primary process thinking. Freud held that the primary processes were predominant in the thinking of very young children, in dreams, psychological symptoms, and hallucinatory states, as well as functioning as an ever-present unconscious influence on mature thinkers. Once someone has reached maturity it is hard to find a pure-culture example of the primary processes— our rational, category-based secondary processes are always actively attempting to reinterpret and understand the primary processes in secondary process terms (see Chapter 4). However let me now present aspects of the case of Mrs M, a patient showing much evidence of primary process thinking during her treatment for acute schizophrenia during her stay on the inpatient psychiatry unit of the University of Michigan Hospitals in 1976.

A case with primary processes much in evidence

In the throes of an acute psychotic episode, suffering greatly with obvious delusions in a hallucinatory state, Mrs M, screamed in pain and shouted several times: "This delivery is killing me. It's the head and shoulders. It is killing me." Simultaneous with this repeated plaintive utterance, she tried to forcefully push a hard plastic bottle of "Head and Shoulders" shampoo against her pelvis. At the time of this hallucination Mrs M was 55 years old. She was the mother of several grown children all of whom she had delivered normally decades before. But just prior to this hospitalization Mrs M had been told of an advanced gynecological malignancy that would require surgery. This was the likely precipitating cause of the acute exacerbation of her chronic psychotic condition.

---

[5] For more on the nature of the primary processes see Brakel (2002).

Her hallucination/delusion—that she was in some manner giving birth to something—even so roughly described, was clearly a contentful (representational) mental event. Although not in accord with organization by the categories, Mrs M's associations (behavioral and verbal) made it evident that she was experiencing *something* and that her mental faculties were actively representing *something*. Mrs M's associative connections were idiosyncratic; not necessarily consistent, or repeatable even within the context of her psychosis. Further, under the Kantian categories no such object-ish entity—like the funny *object* conjoining the name of the shampoo with past representations of delivering the heads and shoulders of her newborns—could be formed; nor could the pain of childbirth long past be conflated with and combined in one representation with current tumor pain and the pain self-inflicted with a hard plastic item. Indeed, after finally responding to an antipsychotic medication, Mrs M herself no longer made such combinations; her mental contents returned to organization by the categories. It seems then that a different organizational principle, one better able to account for the psychotic content, is needed. It turns out that an associationist principle of combination could work; and owing to some of the very same reasons (to be elaborated in the section below) that Kant found associationism unsuitable to ground (mature, awake) normal human experience.

Kant's negative argument: The case against the associationist principle as grounding (mature normal) human experience

Interestingly as we shall see below, it is Kant's case *against* an associationist law as a grounding for normal, awake, mature mental experience that leads us to the case *for* an associationist law both as grounding "unusual" human experiences (e.g. those in dreams, hallucinations, and young children's thoughts); and as being necessary for the later operation of the category-based principles of synthesis.

Kant was looking for a principle whereby combinations of sensory inputs and part representations are put together determinately to form spatiotemporally integrated, discrete objects. The law of association is a natural candidate, but one Kant dismissed contending that this principle allowed representations to be placed "in any order … [which] would not lead to any determinate connection of them, but only to accidental collocations" (A121). Kitcher (1990) elaborates Kant's view:

> The law of association … links cognitive states related by spatiotemporal contiguity. So, for example, it would connect cognitive states produced by striking matches and

> flames and cognitive states produced by observing different parts of telephones. Only in the second case, however, do *we* [my *italics*] unite those cognitive states in the representation of an object. [But] The law of association operates in the same way in all cases and so could not explain how we achieve different types of representations ... spatiotemporal contiguity is too promiscuous. (p. 79)

And indeed, one can see that associative connections are not only promiscuous but idiosyncratic too. Mrs M's funny hallucinatory/delusional *objects* were put together owing to connections with very specialized meanings to her.

But one need not be hallucinating. Assume that neither Kitcher nor I hallucinate when we have cognitive states produced by striking matches. But maybe my most prominent associative connections to striking matches will be different from Kitcher's. For me now, for example, striking a match is immediately and strongly associated with a sulfur smell and not with flames. And for that matter, in the case of telephone parts, today, when my strongest associates are in the spatial dimension, I might align telephone parts with telephone tables; whereas tomorrow when my temporal associations predominate I might unite telephone parts with telephone rings. Some rather unwieldy funny *objects* could result from combining representations this way. And indeed this was one of Kant's most important worries. Because associationist law could yield these funny subjective *objects* instead of singularly determinate objects spatiotemporally aligned, Kant considered the associationist law unconstrained and incapable of delivering the determinate combinations he sought.

Having dismissed the laws of association as the *a priori* organizing principle of combination, Kant needed an alternative. And he sought "a relation [of representations] which is *objectively valid*, and so distinguished from a relation of the same representations that would have only subjective validity—as when they are connected by the laws of association" (B142, p. 159). For Kant "objectively valid" of course does not and cannot mean representing the thing in itself, a realm of which human cognizers can have no knowledge. Instead "objectively valid" refers to the much more modest ability to achieve the object representations we as a species ordinarily agree upon and are capable of consensually experiencing. For this Kant wanted his *a priori* principle to produce a determinate organization of representations as "they are combined in the object, no matter what the state of the subject might be" (B142, p. 159).

Kant's positive case for priority of an associationist principle

The clearest statement of Kant's positive account of the existence of an associative law, and its necessary anterior position with respect to organization by the categories, comes in the *Prolegomena to any Future Metaphysics* (1783), the work published between the 1781(A) and the 1787 (B) editions of the *Critique of Pure Reason*. Regarding the existence of a grounding associative principle different from the categories, Lewis Beck White, in his editor's introduction to the *Prolegomena* (Bobbs-Merrill edition 1950), paraphrases a segment of sections 14–38 thus:

> Our representations … are organized through the "association of ideas," giving rise to "judgments of perception" which are valid for us only individually, or [they are organized] by the understanding, giving rise to perfectly universal (nonpersonal) "judgments of experience" which are valid for all minds. (p. xvi)

Beck continues (in a footnote): "What is it that makes our experience … [an experience of the] knowledge of *objects*?" The answer is, "Its conformity to rules which are not rules of private association, but rules of synthesis" (footnote 10, p. xvi). Given this, Kant's own words in section 18 (p. 46) do the work of demonstrating the priority of these private subjective associative organizations:

> All of our judgments are at first merely judgments of perception: they hold only for us (that is for our subject), and we do not until afterward give them a new reference (to an object) and desire that they should always hold good for us and in the same way for everybody else.

In other words—first there are representations as they go together for me subjectively; and then there are representations as they go together "objectively" irrespective of how they might be put together idiosyncratically by me.

The necessity of an anterior associationist synthetic principle

Mrs M: After the acute psychotic episode

In order to demonstrate the necessity of an associationist combinatory principle anterior to organization by the categories, let us first return briefly to Mrs M's story. While Mrs M was hallucinating, although the mental contents of the hallucinations/delusions were obviously not organized in accord with the categories, she was actively experiencing and representing *something*. Some sort of associationist law, actively and idiosyncratically applied fits as the organizational principle best able to provide an account for the content of the hallucination/delusion. But what about after the hallucinations; how would Mrs M's experience be characterized then?

Initially we worried that there would be no "after the hallucination" experiences for Mrs M as her hallucinations, delusions, and her acute psychotic state were quite unresponsive to the first line of antipsychotic drug we gave her.

In fact she became increasingly agitated as we increased the dose. This para-doxical reaction required that we switch her to a different antipsychotic agent, which fortunately was quite effective (see Cameron and Wimer 1979). Once this second medication had reached an adequate level in her system, she calmed down. Also, and rather more abruptly than is typical for such patients, she stopped hallucinating and immediately ceased her activities with the shampoo bottle. Soon she talked coherently about her children, her tumor, her upcom-ing surgery, and even the need to shampoo her hair. She also could remember part of her hallucination, particularly how she had conflated the long past pain of giving birth to her children with the current pains of her tumor and that of the plastic "Head and Shoulders" shampoo bottle as she forced it against her pelvis. On the basis of this post-hallucinatory conversation, any Kantian (really anyone) would have characterized Mrs M's no-longer-delusional experiences of the various objects under discussion—the babies being delivered, the sham-poo bottle, the tumor—as good examples of ordinary human experiences of objects. In short, after responding to the medication she once again could, in Kant's words, recognize representations "as they are combined *in the object*, no matter what the state the subject might be" (B142, p. 159).

The associative principle: Kant's negative account, Kant's positive account, and a supposition from Mrs M's case

I will now make the following claim: When we take (1) Kant's argument against an associative principle as a ground for (normal mature) human experience in conjunction with (2) his positive account of an associative principle of combi-nation preceding categorical synthesis and add (3) a supposition arising from the clinical case of Mrs M, we have the elements we need to argue that an associationist combinatory principle is necessarily anterior to synthesis by the categories. Here is the supposition: some version of the striking cognitive tran-sition obvious in Mrs M as she went from her hallucinatory delusional state to the normal wakeful state *must* have taken place in all of us at a time early in our development before ordinary objects could be differentiated or picked out as such. This *must* be the case if Kant is correct that synthesis by the categories is a combinatory principle in which a determinate organization of representa-tions puts them together as "they are combined in the object, no matter what the state of the subject might be" (B142, p. 159), because (as Kant here implies) for a subject to be able to combine representations as they are in the object no matter what his/her subjective state, this subject on earlier occasions and in less mature states, *must* have put together representations in a fashion such that the subject's own subjective state often did matter. Stated simply, this reading of B142 suggests that subjects cannot bind things together as they are combined in the object without having *contrastive* ground in an earlier and subjective putting together of these representations.

 This account squares well not only with psychoanalytic theory about the primary processes, but also with modern formulations in cognitive neuroscience regarding the development of the capacity for categorizing objects. Edelman (1987, p. 24), for example, states, "at the time of an evolved organism's *first* confrontation with its world, most macroscopic things and events do not, in general, come in well arranged categories." He continues, "Given ... the absence of immutable categories of things ... (p. 26)," particularly in what he characterized as the initially "unlabelled world" (p. 7), we should not be surprised that for many organisms (including humans) "overall 'object distinction' [is] not necessarily veridical" (p. 257).[6, 7] Indeed, cognitive neuroscientists who embrace this view seem to recognize not only that various representations must be put together actively to form an object, but further that experiencing objects objectively constitutes a developmental achievement. Experiencing objects objectively entails distinguishing "veridical" objects from a background of non-objects, not relevant objects, and from objects that are "not necessarily veridical," that is, objects that are subjectively constructed *objects*.

Conclusion

If Kant's transcendental argument for synthesis by the categories is sound, so is the proposition that prior combination by an associative law is necessary. This is the case because synthesis by the categories is dependent upon contrast with

---

[6] In the original Edelman has parentheses around the phrase "not necessarily veridical."

[7] The proposed account *could* also fit (albeit somewhat paradoxically) with the findings of current day developmental psychologists. Spelke and colleagues (see e.g. Baillargeon 1987; Spelke 1990; Spelke and Hermer 1996) have conducted many experiments with children as young as three to five months old, concluding that these babies do regard objects as solid and permanent, with the same boundary features as adults. These findings have been replicated and have increasingly become the accepted view. While this seems to provide evidence against my claim, there is the fact that even at three months of age these children have already had a lot of experience interacting with the post-uterine world. In other words there has been time for the contrast between *objects* associatively and subjectively constructed and those constituted in the usual objective way. And what about those children who are not yet able to perform the object-recognizing tasks that the experimenters have in mind? Presumably, these even younger infants, may be humans who do not yet organize their sensory inputs from various modalities to yield representations immediately fitting together to form the coherent, consistent, repeatable "objective" objects of adult consensual experience. (See Spelke 1983; Gentner 1988; Smith 1989.)

an earlier associative organization. While this may break no new philosophical ground, in highlighting this less than famous aspect of Kant's philosophy of mind, "unusual" human experiences like dreams, hallucinations, and the mentation of the very young, can be shown to be grounded in an associative organizational principle. This has important implications for psychoanalysis. These "unusual" human experiences are of course familiar to psychoanalysts in practice. Moreover, they have been characterized in psychoanalytic theory as consisting of primary process mentation, a type of mentation posited by Freud as distinct from our ordinary waking rationality. Thus the grounding of these types of "unusual" human experiences within the framework of Kant's philosophy of mind is welcome for psychoanalysis because psychoanalytic theory, like other theories, can ever benefit from convergent support from domains not sharing the same assumptions and posits. Equally important, aspects of Kant's philosophy of mind—the categories famously necessary for rational human experience, and the less famous but also necessary and *anterior* associationist organizations required for "unusual" human experiences—have been shown to have application in Freud's theory of mind and in psychoanalytic clinical observations.

Chapter 4

Why primary process is hard to know

This chapter explores a powerful force—the force with which ordinary, secondary process, within-the-categories, rational thought strives to reorganize all primary process mediated mentation in order to experience it as ordinary and mostly rational. Dream content will be used as a common example, as I describe the fate of the dream after awakening. Here I suggest that there are stages in knowing the dream elements as the dream is (a) first dreamt, (b) subsequently remembered, and (c) recounted to oneself and then to another (e.g. the analyst). I maintain that these stages proceed from primary process content outside Kant's categories to secondary process content fully determined by the categories.[1]

The fate of the dream after awakening

Dream formation

Freud (1900) in the *Interpretation of Dreams* presents a remarkably original, extensively argued account of what dreams are and how they are constructed. For Freud, dream contents are essentially constituted by wishes. He posited that at the very core of each dream is a set of wishes presented as fulfilled, and he termed these the "latent dream thoughts." In ordinary rational secondary process form, these latent dream thoughts simultaneously represent a combination of both current day conflictual wishes and, perhaps more importantly, forbidden infantile wishes, and represent them in a special way—as totally fulfilled, exactly as desired by the dreamer. And yet, Freud was quite aware that most "manifest" dreams do not transparently present such wishes as fulfilled—certainly not in any rational, straightforward, secondary process fashion. This made sense to Freud, because despite what he understood as a relaxation of the "censorship" during sleep (something currently explained on the basis

---

[1] The main idea for this chapter originated in Brakel 1984.

of prefrontal lobe disinhibition), the raw, self-serving desire to gratify the forbidden wishes that comprise the latent dream thoughts would be exactly the sort of content that even a weak censoring capacity would not tolerate. To illustrate, take a patient, Mr X, who has always felt eclipsed by his younger sister, Z. As a young boy he hated her, and he can remember wishing to kill her. Now he has a warm adult relationship with her. Meanwhile he has a younger female colleague, also named Z, with whom he has had a moderately good work experience. Now suppose that Mr X's colleague, Z, has just been promoted, and ahead of him. We might expect Mr X to have a latent dream thought with the content: "Z is no longer ahead of me; I've shot her, I've killed her, I've defeated her!" And we would expect that (usually) this sort of thought, representing an unacceptable (although rational) wish as fulfilled, would not be plainly represented in the manifest dream; Mr X's conscience (superego) would not allow it. So what sort of content would be represented in the manifest dream and how would this content represent the latent dream thoughts?

This problem with Mr X's dream illustrates the larger dilemma for Freud the theorist: He claims that the contents of dreams are representations of wishes fulfilled; and yet the secondary process rational contents of the latent dream thoughts—gratified forbidden wishes—cannot be allowed to be represented as such. How can this seeming contradiction be resolved? Freud's innovative solution involves what he termed the "dream-work." Consisting of primary process mechanisms including *displacement, condensation, part-for-whole categorization, symbolism, plastic representability*, and *secondary revision/ elaboration* (each to be described below), the dream-work functions to disguise the secondary process latent dream thoughts such that they can be expressed in the "manifest dream." Thus the resultant manifest dream content does not conform to secondary process ordinary rational form—it is instead primary process in its nature.

Let us return to our demonstration case, Mr. X. Although as discussed, his conscience would probably not tolerate a manifest dream in which X shot Z and Z is dead. Mr Z could very plausibly report the following sample manifest dream, containing the same content in a disguised fashion:

> I came to work just as Z was being shot through the heart. She wasn't dead the way she certainly would have been, she did not even fall down—she jumped up way above my head. The only thing that happened is that mysteriously her shoes were gone. Meanwhile as Z jumped up another co-worker, who was standing beside Z, fell down. But the bullet was nowhere near him.

We can see *plastic representability* in the whole visual structure of the manifest dream and particularly in the way that the new corporate hierarchy is shown as Z "jumps above X's head." One obvious *displacement* is that Z, the current day colleague, stands in for sister Z. In this example we see both a displacement in time and in person. Another example of displacement is that someone else, someone who is not X, shoots Z. Finally a displacement in place can be seen as the physically adjacent colleague falls—not Z. *Condensation* combines the two Zs who cause X trouble, also amalgamating the infantile and current problematic situations. As far as *part-for-whole categorization* (a typical kind of primary process categorization—see Brakel *et al.*, 2000, 2002; Brakel 2004), the childhood Z is classified with the current day Z on the basis of two incidental features or parts—the same name and the fact of getting ahead of X. And if we bring in *symbolism*, whereby Z's shoes stand for her feet, we can also appreciate an additional and important part-for-whole categorization—namely that Z has been left without her shoes, that is, "defeeted" and thereby defeated.

The remembered dream

Regarding the sample dream of Mr X, I have not yet said anything about *secondary revision/elaboration*. I will do so now after a brief comment about the tricky matter of separating the dream-as-dreamt from the dream-as-remembered, a matter relevant to the operation of this final dream-work mechanism. The content of dreams-as-dreamt can only be known as reflected by the content of dreams-as-remembered in the awake state. (Awakening with merely the sense of having had a dream clearly provides even less information, as does the sense of dreaming while still in the dream state.) True, the criteria for counting as a remembered-dream can be fairly lenient—for example, the memory of it can be temporary; one need not even remember it sufficiently to articulate it to someone else—but there is no escaping the fact that because the remembered dream is our only source of information about the content of dreams-as-dreamt, our knowledge of the latter is necessarily limited and possibly skewed.

So how does this all pertain to *secondary revision/elaboration* and what is this mechanism anyway? In the formation of the manifest dream, the primary process mechanisms of the dream-work disguise the secondary process latent dream thoughts such that the resultant manifest dream shows much primary process content; content that is *not* organized in an ordinary secondary process fashion. Thus, in Mr X's sample manifest dream there is no cause and effect or it functions very strangely. Z, for example, does not die from a gunshot wound to the heart, nor does she even fall down; she rises up. Identity too seems odd, and anything but singular—although it is Z who is shot, it is an adjacent co-worker who falls. But note that given even such glaring examples of the absence of usual waking life secondary process organization, Freud reasoned that to form a manifest dream—at least one that can be grasped and remembered as a dream upon awakening—some sort of coherence based on rudimentary secondary process ordering of the primary process dream elements must take place. Here is where the mechanism of secondary revision/elaboration comes in. It functions to construct some overall story that (1) encompasses the disguised latent dream thoughts that have through the dream-work lost their original secondary process coherence, and (2) is at the same time a story itself sufficiently coherent, that is, sufficiently organized according to the formal structures of the secondary processes that the dream can be experienced and remembered as a manifest dream. Said Freud (1913 [1912–1913]) of secondary revision/elaboration, "its purpose is evidently to get rid of the disconnectedness and unintelligibility produced by the dream-work and replace it by a new "meaning." But this new meaning, arrived at by secondary revision, is no longer the meaning of the [latent] dream-thought" (p. 95).

Kantian epistemology and dreams

Looking now at the dream experience in Kantian terms, the dream-as-dreamt, much like a delusion or hallucination, is "an unusual human experience" (using here the terms discussed in Chapter 3). Dreams-as-dreamt are "unusual" in the sense that these experiences cannot be well described by Kant's categories for understanding, nor are these experiences organized by the categories. The primary process contents of manifest dreams and the primary processes formal structures organizing their formation account for the outside-the-category nature of dreams-as-dreamt, much as is the case with delusions and hallucinations.

Let us in fact return to Mrs M, the patient in Chapter 3 who experienced an acute delusional/hallucinatory state so that we can focus on her rapid post-hallucination return to secondary process/Kantian category thinking. Shortly after the administration of an effective antipsychotic medication, Mrs M no longer conflated (1) a Head and Shoulder shampoo bottle with the heads and shoulders of her babies, (2) a tumor growing inside with growing fetuses, nor (3) the pains of delivery with both cancer pain and the pain of forcing a hard plastic bottle against her pelvis. In fact, once she was again in a normal alert awake state, Mrs M not only *did not* condense these objects and events, she *could not*. Mrs M demonstrated a transition from primary process outside-the-categories experiences to those that are secondary process and category-organized. This type of transition can be even better appreciated in the stepwise process by which dreams-as-dreamt in the dream state become dreams-as-remembered in the awake state. This is the case insofar as each step requires secondary process/Kantian category application. For now though, let us look just at the initial stage. Minimally for a dream to be known at all, some activity toward secondary revision/elaboration will have had to take place. If a dream-as-dreamt cannot be organized according to the formal structure of even rudimentary secondary process Kantian categories, it cannot be coherent, remembered, grasped—it cannot be *known*; and the dreamer will likely be left only with a sense of having dreamt but no remembered content. Moreover, as was the case with Mrs M once she returned to an alert waking state, as soon as a dreamer awakens and is in the alert waking state, he/she has no choice but to operate according to the secondary process/Kantian category formal organization dominating adult human thought; he/she thereby *cannot* access the mostly primary process dream-as-dreamt.

In fact as we explore the next stages—from remembering the dream to recounting it—it will become increasingly clear that the force of the secondary processes/Kantian categories toward organizing knowledge is so powerful that primary process manifestations get reconfigured and are themselves increasingly hard to know.

The recounted dream

To recount a dream, even to rehearse it to oneself, but especially to tell it to another, for example, to the analyst, further secondary process/Kantian category organizing is necessary. In Mr X's dream above note that although there is much primary process *content*, the dream is always reported in the *form* of failed secondary process/Kantian category expectations. Thus Z neither dies nor falls despite a bullet to the heart. She instead jumps up as another person falls, even though the bullet did not even graze this second person. Mr X's dream report is thus replete with examples of cause and effect *not* operating. Further there is a *violation* of singular identity as Mr X notes that the bullet fells the wrong person. Finally, Mr X is aware in his report of the dream that normal time and space are *not* in effect as, for example, Z's shoes mysteriously disappear. It is a function of the *secondary revision/elaboration* to organize the primary process dream material such that the dreamer can first remember it, and beyond that recount it. Secondary process/Kantian category formal structures are necessary for such a report. Thus, the primary process dream contents, *impossible* to grasp or remember simpliciter, cannot be recounted unless the secondary process/Kantian category form is imposed as a framework. Dreams where *failed* cause and effect, *failed* singular identity, and *failed* spatial and temporal relations are reported, are indeed dream reports organized in the formal terms of the secondary processes and Kantian categories; these "failures" notwithstanding[2] —there is no other organization specified.[3]

---

[2] This is the case in the same sense that the phrase "not horses" is about horses.

[3] By the same token, it is precisely because the primary process manifest dream must be remembered and recounted in secondary process terms that dreamers often get the sense

So why is primary process hard to know?

Despite its vital importance, I have not yet directly addressed this question. All the elements for an answer, however, are now present, and so I will address the problem forthwith. When one is thinking in a primary process as opposed to a secondary process fashion, with the formal operating principles of the primary processes, reality-testing based on rationality is not possible. Primary process is not rational, does not operate with standard everyday logic, and is not guided by the reality principle.[4] Testing reality—including trying to gain evidence for or against hypotheses, modifying beliefs according to evidence, and even discarding beliefs as beliefs whenever sufficient contrary evidence has accrued—is not something primary process thinkers can do. Thus, primary process thinkers are unable to meet the cognitive requirements necessary to properly hold beliefs, namely the ability to regulate beliefs according to the truth conditions that obtain in the world (see Chapters 5 and 7).[5] Since primary process thinkers cannot have "beliefs-proper," it follows then that they cannot meet the even more demanding cognitive requirements necessary to *know*.[6] Therefore, when primary processes predominate it is hard to know anything, including the primary processes and primary process contents. This is one reason that the primary processes are hard to know.

Beyond this there is another factor. As human beings we are natural-born cognizers and categorizers, beings who not only must know things to live, but who live to know. Human experiences of knowing are organized according to the categories, in a secondary process fashion. Therefore, to participate in the universal human experience of knowing, once we become capable of conscious mentation that is dominated by secondary process—a formal organization of thought suited to rationality, reality-testing, evaluating hypotheses, gaining

that the descriptions of particular dreams are not at all adequate. (See Chapter 6, the section on "Philosophical conclusions," particularly footnote 9, where a related matter is taken up.)

[4] It is a-rational and guided by the pleasure principle. (See Chapters 5, 7, and 8.)

[5] In Chapters 5 and 7, I will in fact argue at length that phantasy rather than belief is the main primary process cognitive attitude.

[6] Primary process thinkers (e.g. higher mammals and birds) do have abilities that can be expressed as "know how"—they have procedural knowledge to negotiate the world, survive and reproduce. (See Brakel and Shevrin 2003); what they lack is the capacity to "know that" regarding evaluating truth conditions of propositions. See David Lewis (1988) for an interesting account of the difference between knowing-that and knowing-how. (See also Brakel, forthcoming, for a summary of different sorts of knowledge.)

true beliefs and knowledge—everything, even primary process content, gets reformulated in secondary process/Kantian category formal terms.

Thus it is because (1) primary process thinkers find it hard *to know anything* at all, and (2) secondary process thinkers automatically transform primary process contents into secondary process/Kantian category form, that the primary processes remain epistemologically opaque. This is why primary processes are hard to know.

Addendum: Clinical implications

While it is the case that a dream must be remembered and reported to be brought into a particular psychoanalytic session, the relation between knowledge of a dream in the sense discussed thus far and psychoanalytic knowledge is anything but straightforward.[7]

For example, the dreamer's need to obscure the original latent (secondary process) dream thoughts may continue once he/she is awake notwithstanding the primary process transformations that took place in the dream's formation. In the awake state, primary or secondary process means could be employed to this end. As an example of the latter, returning to Mr X's sample dream above, he could edit the dream as he tells it to his analyst so that it conforms more closely to an ordinary secondary process account, simultaneously and tendentiously rendering the conflictual aspects less accessible. Furthermore, this revising could take place consciously (even if the disguising motive is unconscious) or quite unconsciously. Thus edited, the dream report could look a variety of different ways. For instance, Mr X could alter the important detail of Z's shoes being missing, by instead having her shoes flying off after the shot.

As another type of post-awakening secondary process impediment to uncovering the latent dream thoughts, Mr X could have trouble freely associating to the elements of his dream, sticking to secondary process/Kantian category mediated type comments. Since free associations to dream elements often lead back to central primary process dream contents and these in turn often lead to original latent dream wishes, rigid adherence to secondary process thinking is a common after-awakening resistance to psychoanalytic understanding of the dream.

---

[7] Although not Freud's particular focus in *The Interpretation of Dreams*—his masterpiece was dedicated to using dreams and the dreaming mind as a model for his general theory of mind—Freud (1900) demonstrated throughout this work many complex interactions among the forgetting, remembering, and reporting of dreams, all with respect to gaining of clinical psychoanalytic insight, much of this in colorful detail.

Patients' continued need to disguise forbidden wishes can lead them to employ primary process mechanisms after awakening too. A dream that one remembers having dreamt, can for example, seem so full of noncohering primary process contents that one cannot put it together sufficiently to recount it or even remember it. Also, a dreamer can associate to elements of the dream, but without reflecting on the associations and their meaning in terms of his/her conflicts, taking up an entire analytic session with divergent primary process associations.

On the other hand, operating simultaneously but always at odds with the need to disguise dream wishes and conflicts, is the analytic patient's conscious (and unconscious) motive toward expressing these very same dream conflicts toward increased self-understanding. Regarding every aspect of the dream after awakening there is a motive to express as well as obscure. (See Brakel 1984.) This expressive motive, unlike but coexisting with the ubiquitous central Freudian dream motive—to express as fulfilled, unacceptable, infantile wishes—involves trying to understand and know oneself, including one's unconscious wishes and conflicts. Self-understanding also involves a complex interplay of the primary and secondary processes; both modes of thinking are needed to arrive at new psychoanalytic understanding.

Interestingly, psychoanalysis in its clinical application has no standard form for what constitutes the most efficient route to learning one's conflicts. The general recommendation for "saying what comes to mind"—that is, for freely associating, holds for dreams as it does for other contents; but even here there are small daily paradoxical events. Take for example the following: For a given patient a particular forgotten dream lacking the secondary process structure for remembering and recounting it, may in fact reveal more than if it had cohered sufficiently to be remembered. This can be the case, if for instance, the meaning of the forgetting itself proved quite important. But there is an unavoidable confound: it is of course impossible to compare directly a session in which a certain Dream D was reported, with a session in which Dream D would have been forgotten, and equally impossible to compare a Dream F that was forgotten, with whatever Dream F would have been if remembered and reported. After all one only has either the forgotten dream or the remembered dream. And yet even this statement must be modified some-what, as the dream can be remembered later, or forgotten in the midst of reporting it. As should be obvious, the clinical importance of the fate of the dream after awakening must be determined on a case-by-case, dream-by-dream, and session-by-session basis. Unlike the clear progression in predictable stages that is seen in the epistemology of knowing one's dreams after awakening, there are no clear guidelines toward predicting increased psychoanalytic understanding.

Conclusions

Primary process is hard to know. Primary process thinkers do not evaluate truth conditions. Because they cannot do so, they do not attempt to regulate representations for considerations of truth. And they cannot perform tests of reality. Since knowledge is thus not in the domain of primary process thinkers, for primary process thinkers *everything is hard to know*, including knowing primary process operations and primary process contents.

Humans, however, seek to know. Because virtually all humans develop into predominately secondary process thinkers (at least in terms of conscious mentation), and because secondary process thinkers can evaluate truth conditions, regulate representations according to considerations of truth, and test reality, knowledge *is* possible. And yet primary process remains hard to know because secondary process thinkers forcefully and automatically reformulate and reinterpret all primary process material into a form that is organized in accord with the secondary processes. What drives this powerful force? To my knowledge, no psychologist has ever made the case as strongly as Kant. For Kant, the very possibility for human experience and knowledge necessitates constituting human experience and knowledge according to the categories. Although we cannot know things-in-themselves, what we can *know* consists of the categories themselves and whatever content results from them. Processes and contents outside-the-categories (like primary process operations and their resultant contents) thus for Kant can have no epistemic standing.[8]

Psychoanalytic understanding is a hybrid. Although it depends upon working with "unusual" contents epistemically—as for example the contents of dreams—merely knowing such contents will guarantee nothing in terms of increased psychoanalytic understanding. Instead psychoanalysis, as a clinical method seems to work by privileging both primary and secondary process contents in a technique (free association) that swings back and forth between the formal principles of the primary and the secondary processes. But the clinical technique, its efficacy, and explanations are beyond the scope of this book. Psychoanalytic clinical theory however, does share a vital assumption

---

[8] But see Chapter 3 where "unusual" human experiences are recognized (known), motivating a Kantian-style transcendental argument for outside-the-categories primary processes and their contents.

with the general psychoanalytic theory of mind—one that is at the very core of this book—namely that primary process a-rational thinking is truly representational thought. It is time that I make good my claim to develop a case for primary process a-rational mentation as mentation with true content. Part III, consisting of Chapter 5, follows immediately, and is devoted solely to that very task.

Part III

Something new for the philosophy of mind

Part III is the centerpiece of this book. It consists of an extended argument for the coherence and plausibility of a contested part of psychoanalytic foundational theory—Freud's Corollary One, namely that there exist two systems of mentation with different operating systems, the primary and secondary processes, *and that primary processes too are truly mental and representational*. This part has just one chapter, Chapter 5, which is devoted to demonstrating that the very concept of mental and contentful[1] primary processes is not incoherent despite the fact that the primary processes are indeed not rational, but a-rational.

The most prevalent view in the philosophy of mind is that for a mental state to be contentful it must be part of a holistically rational system of beliefs and desires. This allows and necessitates that successful interpretation of a mental state, based on rational normativity, constitutes and fixes the determinate content of the mental state. No part of this formula will work for a-rational mentation, which is neither rational nor in standard belief/desire form. Clearly, since I am proposing that primary process/a-rational mentation is contentful, I will need to propose another way to deal with the threat of indeterminacy. Primary process mental states, I will argue, can gain sufficient determinacy of content via a proper-function naturalistic account. Here evolutionary success and selective fitness normativity, instead of interpretative success and rational normativity, constitute the determinate content of particular mental states.

---

[1] In this chapter (as with the others in this book) "mental" is used as synonymous with "psychological"; and "contentful" is synonymous with "representational."

In this way, independent both of rationality and the view of interpreters, primary process mentation can be shown to be contentful.

But the case for this view will require something further—a viable proper-function account for primary process mentation—in other words an argument for the view that the primary processes, when functioning properly, enhance the selective fitness success of those using primary process mentation. I will offer such an account, intrinsic to which is the view that properly functioning primary processes take the form of phantasy and wish rather than belief and desire.

This will be dealt with in great detail below. Here I will add that much is at stake in this chapter. Without the coherence of contentful primary process, not only would my small project founder, but also and of much greater moment, Freud's grand project would fail: the very foundation of psychoanalysis rests on the radical idea that there exists unconscious and a-rational mentation that is contentful and meaningful as such. If, on the other hand my arguments go through successfully and it can be shown that the concept of contentful primary process a-rational mentation is coherent, not only will psychoanalysis benefit, but also the philosophy of mind, as its domain would no longer be restricted to just the rational mind.

Chapter 5

Representational a-rational thinking
A proper-function account for phantasy and wish[2]

Introduction: Background

Freud throughout his career as a theorist (and a clinician) often dealt with mental states that are not rational, but instead either a-rational or irrational. As early as 1900, he clearly differentiated such phenomena from those of our usual rational, waking life, claiming that there were actually two types of mentation. The more familiar, everyday type of thinking he termed "secondary process" mentation. The secondary processes consist of mechanisms, states, processes, and contents that largely constitute our rational thoughts. The other type, he termed the "primary processes," and Freud posited that these primary processes predate developmentally and then coexist with the secondary processes. Following Freud's conception, I hold that the primary processes, although clearly mental and intentional with representational content, lack one or more of the hallmarks of the rational. Thus, whereas secondary process rational mentation (1) is tensed (i.e. is about what occurs in a specific real time—past, present, or future), (2) is reality-tested, (3) originates from a single agent's experientially continuous viewpoint, and (4) tolerates no contradictions; primary process mentation demonstrates at least one, often several, and sometimes all of the following: (1) Primary processes are without tenses. They involve no conception of past or future, only a tenseless and unexamined present. (2) In primary process mentation there is no reality-testing—no attempt to regulate representations for considerations of truth. More specifically, no distinctions can be made among what is, what is not but is possible,

---

[2] This chapter with slight revisions first appeared as in Brakel (2002). I thank Ruth Millikan for her reactions to this material and David Velleman for reading and discussing many earlier versions.

and what cannot be. (3) Primary processes do not originate from an agent's experientially continuous viewpoint. They operate at a developmental level at which there is yet to be a stable self, capable of grasping (in any fashion) continuity-in-experience—this being a minimal requisite for 'self' to stand out against the protean background of not self. (4) Standard logic is not employed in primary processes. Most notably, contradictions are tolerated.[3]

Having set out some basic characteristics of primary process mentation, I want to make clear that the goal of this chapter is not to argue for or against its existence.[4] Rather, I am arguing for the *coherence* of the notion of the primary processes as mental states with content.[5] For the mere concept of primary processes as contentful but nonrational already raises a critical issue upon which two important contemporary views in the philosophy of mind diverge. The first of these views, that of attributionism, would deny the possibility of mentation that is a-rational yet representational. For attributionists of every stripe—certainly for Donald Davidson (1970b, 1973, 1974, 1975, 1982) the most extreme adherent, but no less for the moderates, Daniel Dennett (1978, 1987), Richard Cherniak (1981), and Stephen Stich (1983)—mental contents are to be determined by interpretations based on attributing and then assuming holistic rationality. Insofar as attributionism holds that mentation must be interpretable in order to be contentful, and must be largely rational to

---

[3] As surprising as the fourth feature might seem, it can be seen to follow from any one of the other three primary process characteristics mentioned (and of course any combination thereof). If one lacks the capacity to grasp one's own experiences as having continuity for example, there is no unitary agent holding both X and a contradiction of X to be true. Likewise, and even more basically, before attempts to regulate representations for considerations of truth, any proposition that is considered merely "is". While an external view would regard this as a default consideration-as-true, from the internal viewpoint there is no attempt or even capacity to get the truth conditions right. This being the case, take some X that "is" (i.e. is considered-as-true); but if a contradiction of this X is also considered in this manner, prior to considerations of truth and falsity, this ~X "is" (i.e. is considered-as-true) no less. Finally, tenselessness too can yield tolerance for contradiction. If every moment is an unexamined timeless present, a "now" with no history and no future, X held at moment t will not be negated by ~X being held at $t+1$, nor will the ~X of moment $t+1$ be negated when at $t+2$ X is held. I thank Jennifer Church (personal communication) for this final point.

[4] In a series of papers based on empirical experiments using non-psychoanalytic measures to index primary process responses, I do argue for the existence of the primary processes. I base my conclusions on convergent evidence as I find an increase in primary process responses just where psychoanalytic theory predicts. (See Brakel 2004; Brakel *et al.*, 2000, 2002; Brakel and Shevrin 2005.)

[5] Content should be understood in the usual way. I am not holding for any special, new "primary process" type content.

be interpretable; this view would prevent the theory of primary processes from getting off the ground.

The first goal of this chapter is to refute the attributionism objection. I will do this by presenting an alternative account that can accommodate the primary processes as contentful, without losing ground to the problem of indeterminancy. The alternative account is Ruth Millikan's proper-function naturalism. Millikan's view can be understood as adopting a different normative assumption from that of the attributionists' assumption of interpretable holistic rationality. Millikan's program makes the normative assumption of selective success utilizing evolutionary explanation. This undermines the attributionist claim that mental content is contentful exclusively in virtue of being rational and thereby interpretable, and opens the way for contentful states that are a-rational.[6] But to complete the Millikan-style proper-function naturalistic case for a-rational primary process contentful states, a viable proper-function explanation for the primary processes must be added. Indeed, then, the second goal of this chapter is to provide just such a proper-function account for these a-rational aspects of human mentation.

The attributionism objection

Attributionism, even in its mildest version, poses serious problems for the primary processes in two ways: (1) Attributionists base the ascription of mental content upon an assumption of rationality. (2) Attributionists take up only two types of propositional attitudes, *belief* and *desire* (or some attitude functioning as such), as the units of interpretation. The first feature of the view is a problem because primary processes are by definition contentful states that are not rational. The second feature is a problem because primary processes *cannot take the form of belief.* Given that primary process mentation is marked by no reality-testing, in fact no attempt to regulate representations for considerations of truth, beliefs cannot be among the propositional attitudes that comprise the primary processes. This is the case because beliefs are precisely those propositional attitudes which aim to get their truth-values right. Clearly those desires figuring into such interpretations—those desires predicated upon beliefs in order to get fulfilled—will also not be a suitable vehicle for primary processes.[7] But another pair of propositional attitudes, *phantasy* and *wish,*

---

[6] I will use a-rational rather than irrational. Irrational implies the rational gone wrong. A-rational refers instead to states not-yet rational and not-yet irrational.

[7] Other sorts of desires can consist in primary process contents. (See Chapter 8.)

does admit of primary process content.[8] I will take up primary process content in these latter proposition types in a section below (see pp. 74–77).[9]

The basic tenets of attributionism can be seen most clearly in Davidson's work.[10] Thus minimal attributionism holds that (1) content is constituted only when content can be attributed, (2) for content to be attributed, interpretable beliefs must be ascribed, and (3) belief ascription can take place only in the context of holistic rationality. (Regarding these three points see especially Davidson 1974a, p. 237, 231 and Davidson 1973, p. 259.)

Before I attempt to undermine the attributionism objection to the very notion of primary processes, I want to point out that the fundamentals of attributionism have some appeal. It is the attributionists, and Davidson in

---

[8] Note that not all philosophers writing on psychoanalytic theory agree with my view on primary process propositional attitudes. In fact, the view presented here may be unique. Sebastian Gardner (1993) in *Irrationality and the Philosophy of Psychoanalysis* and Jonathan Lear (1998) in *Open Minded* regard primary process attitudes as pre-propositonal. From the opposite direction, Marcia Cavell (1993) in *The Psychoanalytic Mind: From Freud to Philosophy* considers the manifestations of primary process contents comprising propositional attitudes as proto-rational, proto-secondary process. (See Chapter 9 for more on the views of Gardner, Lear, and Cavell contrasted with those presented in this book.)

[9] See also Brakel (2001), "Phantasies, Neurotic-beliefs, and Beliefs-proper." It is conceded that the a-rational primary processes cannot be subject to belief/desire interpretations. However, it is not conceded that contentful states are constituted only in virtue of satisfying explanations predicated on belief/desire interpretations. As will be argued below, contentful states can also be constituted in propositional attitudes of the form phantasy/wish.

[10] The views of Davidson to be presented in this chapter are representative of what is basic to attributionism. Other attributionists change certain features of the attributionist program without really changing what is at the core. Cherniak (1981), for example, relaxes the criteria for what counts as rational. Dennett (1987, p. 98) agrees with Cherniak. Stich (1983), a projectivist, suggests that projecting one's own beliefs and mental contents will provide less stringent rationality requirements than assuming rational contents in others. And yet these relaxed-criteria versions of rationality all amount to rationality-attributing nonetheless. Hence, they pose the same difficulties for the *a-rational* primary process.

Davidson is however the most extreme attributionist with respect to his other views, not to be taken up here. Perhaps most striking are his claims on what it takes "to have a belief." He (1975, p.170) says that "Can a creature have a belief if it does not have the concept of belief? … it cannot…. Someone cannot have belief unless he understands the possibility of being mistaken, and this requires grasping the contrast between truth and error—true belief and false belief." Clearly these requirements limit those to whom Davidson will ascribe beliefs to humans, and rather mature humans at that. Dennett (1978, p. 271), at the other pole, counts as a believer any "system whose behavior can be … explained and predicted by relying on ascriptions to the system of *beliefs* and *desires*."

particular, who, for example, have cogently maintained that the very concepts of a-rational, irrational, and inconsistent mental content states *depend* upon a background of rational mental states against which they can be contrasted. Thus in his essay "Mental Events" Davidson (1970b) states:

> Crediting people with a large degree of consistency cannot be counted mere charity: it is unavoidable if we are to be in a position to accuse them meaningfully of … some degree of irrationality. Global confusion… is unthinkable, not because imagination boggles, but because too much confusion leaves nothing to be confused about. (p. 221)

But what sort of dependence is Davidson really implying here? Certainly it seems incontrovertible that even Freud's initial *recognition* of the concepts of inconsistent, irrational, and a-rational human mental states depended on the contrasting background of consistent and rational human mental states. But this epistemologic dependence is more modest than the ontologic dependence Davidson holds. For him, unless a subject can be shown to have a holistic background of consistency and rationality, belief ascription will not be possible; hence mental content will not be attributed. Then, because mental content attribution is what constitutes mental content, not only will the mental content of that subject remain unknown—*there will be no mental content* for this subject at all. Note that by these criteria children under the age of around three years, primates, adults in dream-states, and certainly mammals in other orders, and so on, will lack mental content states.

Still Davidson does acknowledge the existence of (what he must regard as infrequently occurring) irrational mental states. Holding in his essay "Paradoxes of Irrationality" that "irrationality appears only when rationality is evidently appropriate" (1982, p. 299), he wants to extend his view of mental content to account for the irrational-but-mental. That this effort might prove problematic, he admits, stating that on the one hand, if he explains irrationality too well, he fears he will have reduced the phenomenon to rationality. Yet on the other hand, if he finds that what is irrational is merely incoherent, then irrational phenomena will cease to be recognizable as mental, and will thereby on his view (in which the epistemic is constitutive) cease *to be* mental at all.

Nonetheless Davidson (1982) fashions a compromise solution with the use of what he considers some psychoanalytic, Freudian-style concepts. For Davidson, human agents are capable of irrational acts owing to a split in "mental structures" into two or more semi-autonomous mental structures. Some of these semi-autonomous structures can even be unconscious. What is vital for Davidson, whether a structure is conscious or unconscious, is that each such semi-autonomous unit is an internally coherent *rational system of beliefs and desires*, where *within each such structure* psychological *reasons are rational causes*.

Between different structures, on the other hand, there are *nonrational causes*. These nonrational casual relations between different structures (and between the contents of the different structures) produce and account for irrationality. (Davidson 1982, pp. 290–304).[11]

While Davidson does believe in a sort of Freudian unconscious—a semi-autonomous unconscious structure containing beliefs and desires that are irrational in relation to an agent's conscious attitudes—it is a Freudian unconscious much colored by Davidson's own attributionism. The unconsciously sequestered mental contents are for Davidson not only rational within their own semi-autonomous unit, they comprise an internally consistent *rational system of beliefs and desires*. Thus here no less than elsewhere, attributionism precludes Freud's notion of the primary processes, in which the primary processes, whether conscious or unconscious, are neither rational, nor in the form of beliefs and their associated desires. Moreover, while the concept of the unconscious for Freud was not static over his long career as a theorist, it certainly can be said that at no time did he characterize the unconscious as a coherent system of rational (secondary process) beliefs and the desires predicated upon them.[12]

Irrational and a-rational states occurring more than just very infrequently would, from Davidson's position, allow too many interpretative hypotheses—in other words, indeterminacy would threaten. His principle of charity argument, central to his attributionism,[13] clearly arises from this threat. At first Davidson's argument for the principle of charity seems to aver to the need for *some* normative constraint to narrow the domain of eligible interpretations. Davidson (1967, p. 27) states in "Truth and Meaning" that "we must maximize the self-consistency we attribute to him [an alien], on pain of not understanding *him*. No single principle of optimum charity emerges; the constraints

---

[11] Also, as long as intra-structural causal relations between states (belief/desire or belief/belief) are most often rational, Davidson does allow that nonrational causal connections occasionally take place intra-structurally between states. However as Jennifer Church (1987) points out, this strategy cannot help Davidson account for the systematic, consistent, even predictable nature of much irrationality.

[12] In fact contradictions even within a particular psychological state, like a phantasy, are much more typical of the Freudian view. For examples of such contradictions internal to a phantasy, see Chapter 7.

[13] Davidson's principle of charity argument appears in many places in addition to those that I have cited. See, for example, "Thought and Talk" (1975, particularly p. 159), in *Truth and Interpretation* (1984). And see, "Mental Events" (1970b, particularly pp. 221–3), and "The Material Mind" (1973, particularly pp. 257–9), both in *Action and Events* (1980).

therefore determine no single theory [of meaning]." And again in "Belief and the Basis of Meaning" (1974b, p. 154) without mentioning rationality, he stresses that, "Each interpretation and attribution of an attitude is a move within a holistic theory, a theory necessarily governed by concern for consistency and general coherence with the truth." (Both of these essays are in the *Truth and Interpretation* (1984) collection.) But it becomes clear that Davidson is really holding for only one type of normative constraint—the charitable attribution of holistic rationality. In "Psychology as Philosophy" (1974a, p. 231) he states that we charitably and "necessarily impose conditions of coherence, rationality, and consistency." Later (p. 237) he adds that "if we are intelligibly to attribute attitudes and beliefs, or usefully describe motions as behaviour, then we are committed to finding, in the pattern of behaviour, belief, and desire, a large degree of rationality and consistency." Still later (p. 239) he states that "The constitutive force in the realm of behaviour derives from the need to view others, nearly enough, as like ourselves"—that is, "mostly rational." Finally, in yet another essay, "On the Very Idea of a Conceptual Scheme" (also in *Truth and Interpretation*) one can see that for Davidson the notion of *some* charitable principle for providing normative constraint has collapsed into his particular choice of rational normativity charitably ascribed. He writes (1974c, p. 197): "charity is not an option, but a condition of having a workable theory…. Charity is forced on us; whether we like it or not, if we want to understand others, we must count them right [rational] in most matters."

Davidson's charitable assumption of holistic rationality successfully deals with the indeterminacy problem in an appealing fashion. But is Davidson's normative rationality constraint the only normative constraint that can address indeterminacy? In what follows I will show that Millikan's view embodies a far different normative constraint against indeterminacy, but one no less effective. In Millikan's program evolutionary success supplants rationality success as the normative principle charitably attributed. Contents are determinate not necessarily owing to consistent coherent rationality, but rather insofar as the proper function of such contents can occasion selective reproductive fitness. There is still a pattern to behavior, a consistency and coherence,[14] and there is still the charitable assumption that other beings are like us—it is just that they

---

[14] Note that both the attributionist view and the proper function view fit well with the first two assumptions of psychoanalysis—psychic continuity and psychic determinism. Both of these philosophical programs for fixing content, although using very different laws, assume patterns to behavior, consistency, and coherence, in other words, lawful regularity in these phenomena of interest.

are like us in that selective fitness normativity, rather than rational normativity, allows the possibility of a-rational as well as rational content.

Undermining the attributionism objection

Central to the core of attributionism is the claim that for a mental state to be interpreted as contentful it must be part of a holistically rational system of beliefs and desires—even if the rationality is charitably assumed. Attributionism thereby poses a serious objection to the primary processes as conceptualized by Freud. The primary processes are a-rational by definition—no amount of charity will change this; and the primary processes do not take the form of beliefs and desires predicated upon beliefs. So how can the primary processes be interpreted as contentful?

An answer to this question, which entails refuting the attributionism objection, is the focus of this chapter. The answer comes in two parts. First I will claim, that contrary to the attributionist exclusivity claim for mental contents being determinately interpretable only as they are rational, the primary processes as conceptualized by Freud can in principle be accommodated by another contemporary view of mental content, the naturalist proper-function view of Ruth Millikan. In Millikan's account the indeterminacy problem is solved with a different normativity constraint—the assumption of adaptive and selective fitness success, which neither precludes nor requires rationality. However, within Millikan's program there is an additional step needed to secure the argument that the primary processes are interpretable in terms of selective success and as such contentful. This addition is a proper-function explanation for the primary processes. Second, I will propose just such an explanation for primary processes with a proper-function account of phantasy and wish, an attitude pair analogous to belief and desire but mediated by primary process.

I shall proceed with a review of Millikan's position.

Millikan's proper-function account of representation

To appreciate fully the Millikan view (see Millikan 1993, chapters 3–5, and 9, pp. 51–121 and 172–92) it is useful to look at her concepts of proper function and Normal conditions as they apply to simpler organ mechanisms and states. The function of sweat glands is to secrete sweat. But with regard to "proper function," this is only part of the story. For the sweat glands to be indeed properly functioning, "Normal" conditions for the sweat secretion are required. Thus the condition of the body being overheated, followed by sweat secretion, leading to the body's return to its regular temperature are among the Normal conditions under which sweat gland secretion can be considered to be properly functioning. On the other hand, if there is a tumor at the temperature-sensing center, such that a regular or even a low temperature leads to sweat gland secretion, even though the sweat glands themselves are fully operative, they are not functioning under Normal conditions. As Millikan (1993, p. 73) says, "though it is a proper function of the sweat glands to secrete sweat, this is so [Normally] if and when the body is overheated." Now this distinction is important because only organisms with sweat glands properly functioning *under Normal conditions*, and not organisms with merely adequately function-ing sweat glands, were (and are) aided in their proliferation in part because of these properly functioning sweat glands. In other words, the Normal condi-tions are those conditions under which the inherited proper function confers the selective advantage.

Turning now to belief-manufacturing mechanisms, their function is to manufacture beliefs. But quite like the case above, only organisms with prop-erly functioning belief-manufacturing mechanisms *under Normal conditions* were (and are) aided in their proliferation in part because of these properly functioning belief-manufacturing mechanisms. Belief-manufacturing mecha-nisms function to produce beliefs, but not all beliefs are properly functioning under Normal conditions. Normal conditions, those that conferred (and confer) selective fitness, are those in which the truth conditions of the representation (belief) match those obtaining in the world. Thus only mechanisms manufac-turing these true beliefs are those belief-manufacturing mechanisms that are properly functioning under Normal conditions. In Millikan's words (1993, p.73):

> [I]t is a proper function of the belief-manufacturing mechanisms in John to produce beliefs-that-*p* only if and when *p*, for example beliefs that Jane is in Latvia only if and when Jane is in Latvia…. To turn this around, a belief that Jane is in Latvia is, and is *essentially*, a thing that is not Normally in John unless Jane is indeed in Latvia.

But note that for Millikan there is nothing *a priori* or necessary in believers holding true beliefs, or in coming by these beliefs rationally. Rather, true beliefs and the rationality they usually entail are contingently determined biological norms. The Normal conditions for beliefs—those conditions that confer selec-tive advantages to belief holders—are those in which the truth conditions of the belief's representation are constituted by the truth conditions of the world. But, it just happens to have been the case (and presumably continues to be so) that our ancestors capable of having these rationally mediated true beliefs, and exercising this capacity enough of the time, had selective advantages such that the mechanisms supporting rationally mediated true belief generation were reproduced.

Actually, Millikan's view on rationality could not be more different from that of the attributionists. For the attributionists it is the rational which provides the underpinnings for intentionality and mental representation. Millikan (1993, p. 109) paraphrases the serious attributionist worry concerning her view thus: "How could anything exhibit intentionality... that was not, at least to an approximation, rational? Is not rationality, as Dennett claims, 'the mother of intention'..."[15] Millikan's various comments on toads and lead pellets can be used to address this worry in two steps. First, she can show that by her criteria toads, even though they cannot differentiate lead pellets from bugs—owing to a powerful reflex mechanism they will swallow countless numbers of both kinds, have contentful representations of bugs. She (1993, p. 94) explains that "a certain kind of small, swift image on the toad's retina, manufactured by his eye lens, represents a bug, for that is what it must correspond to if the reflex it (invariably) triggers is to perform its proper function normally." In other words, at time t when the image corresponds to a bug and not a lead pellet, the toad's representation producer properly functions and produces a properly functioning, that is, fitness-enhancing representation of a bug. At time $t+1$ when the new image corresponds to a lead pellet, the toad's representation producer still functions properly and a bug is represented again—but this time the representation is not a properly functioning one, for abNormal conditions (namely that lead pellets are present but not bugs) have obtained. Only those representations of bugs that have contributed to toad nutrition and thus to toad reproductive success are Normal condition representations. But the representation of bugs when only pellets are present are representations of bugs no less; the difference is these bug (pellet) representations are abNormal condition representations.

In the second step, she can show that she has made no claim whatsoever for toads having rational capacities. Regarding a toad swallowing lead pellets, Millikan (1993, p. 76) holds that "His inner activity does not include separable states or features, one to correspond to his belief that the pellets are bugs, another to his desire to eat bugs." In contrast, she (1993, pp. 76–7) states that with humans

> beliefs are separate entities from desires and... beliefs and desires are things that can interact with other beliefs and desires to form new beliefs and desires. That is beliefs and desires can participate in inference processes.... Indeed... the ability to combine beliefs and desires in novel ways, is surely the essence of rationality.

---

[15] This phrase is from Dennett (1978, p. 19).

With her use of minimalist naturalist criteria Millikan has been able to effectively divorce representations, complete with fixed determinate intentional content, from rationality.[16] Whereas for attributionists,[17] content fixing is owed to ascribing beliefs, assuming (charitably) general rationality, and then success in belief interpretability; Millikan resolves the indeterminacy problem and fixes content in a different way. The truth conditions of a representation are constituted by the Normal conditions for that representation—in other words the particular conditions under which fitness success just happened to be conferred.[18] For Millikan the normative assumption of selective success replaces the normative assumption of rationality success; and her normative constraint narrowly determines the content of representations, resolving the indeterminacy problem with equal success. Thus toads narrowly represent both bugs and lead pellets as "bugs"—the former are Normal representations; the latter abNormal—in Millikan's system toads have no wide, disjunctive indeterminate representation "bug or pellet."

Note that freed of the burdensome charity of presuming holistic rationality, Millikan (1993, p. 91) can state that "it is not necessary to assume that most representations are true. Many biological devices perform their proper functions not on the average but just often enough... it is conceivable that the devices

---

[16] The "divorce" between representations and rationality may not look like a divorce at all, particularly with higher order representations like beliefs, since for Millikan beliefs clearly do participate in rational inference processes. But although Normal condition properly functioning beliefs are rational, that they are rational is purely contingent in the Millikan program. Rational true beliefs just happen to be the sorts of beliefs that have contributed to the selective fitness of their holders. With respect to beliefs then, rather than a married or divorced couple, representation and rationality are more like two people who just happen to be next-door neighbors and find that they actually like one another. For representations that are not beliefs (e.g. toads' representation of bugs), the Millikanian position allows that rationality need not be even contingently related. I will further claim below that there are also even fully propositional contentful states that are quite unrelated to rationality.

[17] William Lycan (personal communication), suggested that Dennett, unlike Davidson, can claim this sort of divorce between rationality and representation too as Dennett's "subpersonal agencies have states with real (nonattributive) intentional content." It seems to me that this is not quite apt, for Dennett's subpersonal agencies while indeed not requiring rationality have only perceptual contents, not contentful propositional states.

[18] Again in the case of human beliefs, the Normal fitness-enhancing conditions are those in which the truth conditions of the representations just do happen to match those of the world.

that fix human beliefs fix true beliefs not on the average, but just often enough."[19] Further, Millikan has no trouble accounting for false representations. A toad representing lead pellets as bugs shows a frequent form of misrepresenting which yields false representations. The analog with people and their beliefs is straightforward. False beliefs and irrational beliefs are beliefs for Millikan no less; and they need not indicate any problems in the mechanisms needed for believing (or even true believing), because false beliefs and irrational beliefs can arise from various abNormal conditions, internal and external. What can be said of false beliefs and irrational beliefs on Millikan's account is that they are beliefs that are incapable of performing their functions in a Normal way. This means they have not been and cannot be the sorts of beliefs that play a role in the selective evolutionary fitness of their believers. On the other hand, rationally mediated true beliefs—only because just enough of these states have had content vital to survival and reproductive success and hence have played a role in their believers' adaptive fitness—are the only beliefs that can be said to be properly functioning under their fully Normal conditions.

Extending Millikan's account to primary process content

Part one: Phantasy and wish, a different pair of attitudes

It is clear that the Millikan view raises no essential or devastating objection to the conception of primary processes as a-rational yet intentional with referring mental content. The Millikan program can be applied to something that is not a rational system like the primary processes; and for Millikan a mental state can be mental without the content having had to result from successful interpretation of rational belief. In fact, given that, for her, successful fixing of mental content is divorced from successful interpretations of rationality—depending instead on Normal conditions toward biological/selective success[20]—primary process mental content could too, if provided with a proper-function account for its use, be accommodated by the Millikanian view.

---

[19] It is presumed that Millikan's biological success criterion for beliefs being true "not on the average, but just enough" is a far less stringent requirement than the attributionist's interpretation success criterion, which demands that most beliefs be true.

[20] Indeed, success in interpreting the rational, vital to the attributionist's program, does not play a role for Millikan. However there is a very different sense in which "interpretation" is involved in the Millikan program, namely in what is seen as constitutive of Normal explanations for biological success. With the typical standards of the philosopher of biology she holds, for example, that Normal explanations are the most simple and proximal explanations. These do indeed constitute rational and interpretative constraints

But before such a proper-function account for the primary processes can be offered, there is one further matter that must be addressed, and this concerns the types of propositional attitudes used in understanding primary process mentation. As alluded to earlier in this chapter, primary process mentation does not take the form of belief and desire. Yet for the attributionists belief and desire constitute the essential attitude pair. No other attitude pair will serve because *belief* plays a unique and central role in the attributionist program. Although Millikan too devotes much attention to belief and desire, nothing in her theory necessitates that this pair plays a core role.

With respect to belief and desire, that they are a natural focus for theorists owes not merely to convention, but instead reflects the readiness with which beliefs and desires lend themselves to intentional and motivational analyses. However, because beliefs by their very nature carry with them a special relationship to truth, beliefs, and the desires dependent on them may not in fact be the appropriate attitude pair upon which to base an understanding of mental contents in general.

Following Velleman (1998, pp. 7–8; 2000, pp. 111–18 and pp. 247–54), it can be seen that many propositional attitudes can be classified as belonging either to the cognitive group—where p is believed-true, supposed-true, hypothesized-true, imagined-true, or phantasized-true, which in each case implies that p is to be in correspondence with the world; or to the conative group—where q is desired-true or wished-true, implying that the world is to be brought into correspondence with q. What differentiates the various cognitive attitudes from one another? One critical point is that belief stands out from all of the others with respect to its relationship to the truth. When I suppose p to be true, I can do this with no commitment whatever to my views on p's truth. For the sake of an argument, discussion or game I can suppose p true, even when I know p to be false. With hypothesizing p true, I do have more at stake; I am betting on p to be true and trying to get p's truth-value right, but admitting that I need more evidence. But with belief there is no equivocating. I cannot believe p to be true unless I am trying to get p's truth-value right, unless I am aiming at the truth. As Velleman (1998) puts it, supposing and hypothesizing involve, "regarding a proposition *as* true irrespective of whether it *is* true, whereas believing involves regarding a proposition as true with the aim of so regarding it only if it really is" (p. 8).

---

upon what can be considered a Normal explanation. But clearly this is a very different level from the attributionists who must interpret each agent on the presumption of his/her holistic rationality.

Now let us look at the other end of the cognitive attitude spectrum. Phantasizing p true is a cognitive attitude with a relationship to truth that is most different from the relationship between belief and truth. When I phantasize p true, as with supposing p true, I have no commitment as to whether or not I take p to be true. But phantazing p true is very different from supposing p true. Whenever I suppose some proposition to be true, although I have no stake in the truth or falsity of that which I suppose, considerations of truth and falsity are integral. Supposing is after all the active choice to suspend existing truth discerning exercises and to just stipulate p as true. With phantasizing p true on the other hand, rather than being actively suspended, considerations of truth and falsity have never been present; they cannot have been suspended because they have played no part in the phantasy. When I phantasize p true not only am I not interested in the truth-value of p, I am not interested in truth-values at all. The capacity to phantasize p true is prior to the capacity to consider truth and falsity, and prior to the capacity to actively engage in exercises aimed at discerning truth.[21]

All of this suggests a developmental sequence in the cognitive attitudes. Supposing p true and hypothesizing p true both require first acknowledging truth and falsity, and then adopting a particular stance about truth and falsity as regards p. In the case of supposing-true, considerations of the actual truth-value of p are suspended and p is just taken to be true. With hypothesizing-true, there is the informed guess that p is true and the call for further evidence. Believing p true requires evaluating p with respect to p's truth or falsity and believing p only if p is evaluated as true. And belief aims at getting this right. Phantasizing p true (and some playful imaginings that p) require only having the propositional content p, and that is all. In phantasizing-true and some types of imaginings-true there are no attempts to evaluate p's truth or falsity and no aims at getting this evaluation right, because there is not yet the capacity to evaluate truth-values or to aim at the truth. So whereas a being must be capable of believing before supposing or hypothesizing is possible, phantasizing and (at least some types of) imagining precede believing. Velleman (1998, pp. 11–12) agrees that "imaging precedes believing in the order of development.... We should therefore conceive of belief as reality-constrained imagining."

This view is not uncontested. Beneath the disagreement, however, lies a common confusion. A confound exists between (1) phantasizings and imaginings

---

[21] The "true" part of phantasizing-true pertains only to the proposition's truth-value as regarded externally, objectively. It does not pertain to the phantasizer's subjective, internal evaluation of truth, as there is none.

that are done without any consideration of truth-values, and are therefore less sophisticated than beliefs, and (2) various instances of fictionalizations and pretendings that, because they require the suspension of considerations of truth, are actually more like supposings and are indeed far more sophisticated than simple beliefs. Note in support of the distinction and the developmental sequence proposed, is the fact that adults are far better than children at devising complex, coherent works of fiction, while children, often "lost" in such playful imaginings, do a much better job of phantasizing that they are trains, elephants, or dinosaurs, or even fast, huge, and hungry "dinosaur-trains."

Again since Millikan's naturalist proper-function view has no intrinsic need to focus on the attitudes of belief and desire, and since there should be no reason in principle that phantasy and wish analyses could not be included, the proper-function account for primary process mentation that I will provide will use the attitude pair phantasy and wish.

Part two: A proper-function account for phantasy and wish

Although phantasizing and believing are both cognitive attitudes with important parallels, they have very different proper functions and very different Normal conditions for the exercise of their proper functions. This is also true for certain individual states of phantasies and beliefs. A Normal condition for the proper function of believing that *p*, and for the proper function of the belief that *p*, is that *p* will be believed-true just in those cases that *p* truly obtains now. It is clear that beings with properly functioning belief mechanisms and belief states have, under this Normal condition, selective advantages.[22] It is owed then to the biological success conferred by the proper function of beliefs *under this Normal condition*, and quite independent of any intrinsic relationship to rationality, that the contents of beliefs are secured. Further, to the extent that the mechanisms for believing and particular belief states continue to function properly *under this Normal condition*, they will presumably contribute to selective fitness and therefore participate in their own proliferation. The particular belief states in which this is best demonstrated are belief states with contents vital for biological fitness. So for example, there are selective advantages for beings who possess not only the general mechanisms for beliefs which will under Normal conditions be true beliefs, but also the particular capacities for Normally true beliefs about the health of conspecifics who are

---

[22] Stephen Stich (1990, see especially pp. 55–70) offers arguments against the assumption that true belief believing enhances selective fitness.

potential mates, the dangerousness of rapidly approaching predators, and the speed of catchable prey.

To understand the parallel situation for phantasizing and particular phantasy states, the promised proper-function account for phantasizing and the phantasies produced is now due. This account begins by stating the proper functions of phantasizing and phantasies. The proper function of phantazing is to produce phantasies, states that I maintain have fixed content in the absence of rationality. Phantasies are properly functioning only when they demonstrate one or more of the four characteristics of primary process mentation enumerated at the beginning of this chapter and summarized as follows. Properly functioning phantasies are (1) without tenses, in other words they are phantasized only in an unexamined present; (2) not reality-tested—they are phantasized without attempts to regulate representations for truth considerations such that, for the agent, phantasies are neither correct nor incorrect; (3) not phantasized from an agent's singular and continuous view point; and (4) phantasized in a manner that the phantasies admit of contradictions and other lapses in ordinary logic.

Having advanced these four proper functions for phantasies, there are two major questions for our proper-function account to address. First, how can the contents of such properly functioning a-rational phantasies be determinately fixed? Second, how can such properly functioning phantasies contribute to the selective fitness of beings that can and do phantasize? Just as the contents of beliefs are fixed by the conditions that are Normal for the proper functioning of beliefs, the Normal conditions for the proper function of phantasies will likewise fix their content. But this can only be the case if under their Normal conditions properly functioning phantasies confer selective fitness advantages for phantasizers. Thus to address both questions I turn now to demonstrating that there are particular conditions under which the proper function of phantasizing and phantasies do confer selective fitness advantages; and as such these Normal conditions will determine and fix the content of the phantasies, quite without rationality.

There are three fitness-conferring conditions for the proper function of phantasy that must be specified, all rather unlike any Normal condition for beliefs:

1) Whereas a fitness-conferring condition for belief is that p will be believed-true now just in cases where p truly obtains now; for phantasy a selective advantage accrues only in the opposite case: that p will be phantasized-true now only in those cases in which p does not now obtain.

2) Although as just indicated one of the fitness-enhancing conditions for the proper function of phantasy p is that p does not obtain now at time t; another condition for the properly functioning phantasy p to confer selective fitness success is that p will obtain later, say at time $t+1$.

3) Finally, the third condition under which the proper function of phantasy *p* provides fitness advantage is that the phantasy with content *p* at time *t* will have afforded some useful practice for the phantasizer, when at time *t*+1, some time after the phantasy *p*, *p* does obtain.

Before I elaborate on these somewhat unusual fitness-enhancing Normal conditions for phantasizing and phantasies, let me square this *proper function under Normal conditions* explanation for phantasizing and phantasies with that of the more familiar proper function Normal explanation for believing and beliefs. With phantasies and phantasizing (as with beliefs and believing) it is not the case that all phantasies will be states derived according to proper function under Normal conditions. Phantasizing *p* to be the case will, for example, be functioning under abNormal conditions, if either *p* does now obtain simultaneous with phantasizing *p̄* at time *t*; or if *p* never obtains in the future.[23] Also (and again parallel to the belief case), only those phantasies functioning properly under Normal conditions will contribute to the selective fitness of the phantasizers, and thereby to reproducing more beings with properly functioning phantasies and the mechanisms supporting them. Finally (and once more as is the case for beliefs), the clearest contributors to selective fitness are those properly functioning Normal condition phantasies whose content is most relevant to vital areas of reproduction and survival, for example, content about the selection of mates, the avoidance of predators and other dangers, and the obtaining of food.

But do we see such phantasies? Yes, we see such phantasies in action during play activity. Many species of birds and mammals, of course including humans, engage in play. Zoologists have observed that play activity is very often of a form that—although it confers no immediate benefits in terms of nutrition, gaining resources, avoiding danger, or attracting conspecifics *now* [24]—does constitute a practice for any or all of these activities, all of which will be very serious business *later*.[25] Thus, human children, young dogs, and in fact many species of mammals play at fighting and they do so with beings who are not enemies. This sort of play, a phantasy lived-out, meets the primary process

---

[23] The fitness-enhancing condition of a phantasy *p* at time *t*, requiring that *p* will obtain later, say at *t*+1, has a Normal condition with an unusual property in that whether or not a particular phantasy *p* is properly functioning under this Normal condition cannot be determined at the time of the phantasy, time *t*. Such determination cannot take place until some time in the future, time *t*+1.

[24] This definition of play activity is from Robert Fagen (1981) in *Animal Play Behavior*.

[25] This is demonstrated convincingly for rhesus monkeys in Symon (1978) in *Play and Aggression: A Study of Rhesus Monkeys*.

criteria necessary to be considered a properly functioning phantasy: X is engaged in "fighting" (of the play-fighting phantasy type) now, at a time when there is no real fighting, with an "enemy," Y, who is no real enemy. Or take three other instances, all with content relevant to biological fitness and all frequently encountered in animals including (with only slight modifications) humans: (1) Z participates in play where Z mock chases mock prey, (2) P pseudo flees from pseudo predators, and (3) R mounts several practice mates, simulating copulation.

All four of these play-phantasy cases meet the criteria (stated above) for primary process proper functioning phantasies: (1) The play-phantasy is engaged in by beings who are unlikely to have a unified continuous experience of their agency. (2) The play-phantasy likely takes place in a tenseless present. (3) Ascriptions of truth and falsity are not applied. (4) The contents are not reality-tested; the mock chases, mock prey, pseudo predators, and practice mates are not real chases, real prey, real predators, or real mates.

But are these properly functioning phantasy-play activities taking place under the fitness-enhancing Normal conditions? The first one is in place: it is not the case that real fighting with a real enemy is going on now. The second and third Normal (selective advantage conferring) conditions for the proper function of phantasies are best considered together. Remember that the second Normal condition specifies that during phantasy p at time t, p does not obtain; but p does obtain later at time $t+1$. And that the third Normal condition further stipulates that when p does obtain later at time $t+1$, conditions will be fully Normal only if the prior phantasy p at time t will have provided the phantasizer a useful practice for p, when at time $t+1$ p then does obtain. Thus as regards X's primary process phantasy-play of today—(1) where X play-fights *now* with those who are non-enemies, (2) where X will *later* actually have to fight real enemies for survival, and (3) where X will fight the real fight more effectively, enhancing survival and reproductive chances, owing to the play-fighting practice—in these cases (and in these cases only) X's primary process phantasies will have been properly functioning under their full Normal conditions.

Given then that (1) there are conditions for the proper function of primary process phantasies which provide selective advantage for beings so phantasizing, and (2) that these conditions can thus be considered as the Normal (although certainly not the typical) conditions for the proper function of primary process phantasies, the content for primary process phantasies can be fixed appropriately,[26] and in the absence of rationality.

---

[26] This analysis, analogous to that regarding beliefs, secures content for those primary process phantasies that are *not* properly functioning and/or *not* operating under

Finally, and very briefly here (but see Chapter 8) let me take up desire and wish. Although these are both conative attitudes and importantly similar, there are significant differences with respect to their proper functions and Normal conditions. About desire Millikan (1993, p. 67) suggests that,

> [T]he most obvious proper function of every desire… is to help cause its own fulfill-ment. For… *the mechanisms in us that manufacture desires*… have proliferated because the desires they produce are sometimes relevant to our flourishing and reproducing, and because relevant desires have sometimes participated in processes that ultimately effected their fulfillment.

In terms of Normal conditions for the fulfillment of desires, Millikan (1993, p. 68) explains that frequently these are not met and consequently desires are often unfulfilled. "Very often the proper functions… are not performed. Indeed, perhaps most desires… are born into a world in which conditions, outer and/ or inner, are not Normal for their fulfillment."

One Normal condition for the proper function of wishes is also to cause their fulfillment. But note the following difference: In order to fulfill a desire, changes in the real world are necessary. These changes often require that beliefs about the real world pertaining to what is desired need to conform to those states of affairs of the real world. Thus if I desire q, a drink of water, and I believe p, that a working water fountain is nearby; my desire for water will likely not be fulfilled by seeking that water fountain, unless my belief that p is correct. Similarly, should I desire to be King of the Hill such that I can then select and keep the best mate, have the choicest food, and scare off predators; the beliefs that (1) in order to do this I must fight with and defeat my rivals, and (2) that I have the power to do so, must conform to reality, if my desire to be King of the Hill is to be met. A wish, on the other hand, needs for its fulfill-ment only that the non-reality-tested world-as-phantasized conforms to what is wished. My wish to be King of the Hill can be fulfilled by different primary process phantasies. I can phantasize that X is King of the Hill and my rival, when X is really not the King and is my friend; and I can have a phantasy of victory over X as we engage in a mock fight. Or, I can phantasize that my current powers are much greater than Z's, the real but far off King of the Hill, and I can continue my phantasy by imagining my successful challenge of Z. Or I can phantasize that Y, who really is fighting Z for the crown, will, after depos-ing Z, bestow the title on me. Hence wishes can be fulfilled far more often than desires. Properly functioning wishes can even have a causal role in producing

---

Normal conditions, much as Normal proper functioning beliefs secure the determinate content of faulty and false beliefs. Note that this analysis allows for the very real possibility that most primary process phantasies are not both properly functioning and Normal.

phantasies in which they will be fulfilled. Clearly desires can have no such proper function role with respect to belief production. However, fulfillment in phantasy is not the only Normal condition for the proper function of wishes. As is the case with phantasies, for wishes to be properly functioning a Normal condition pertaining to the future must be added. Only those wishes which are now fulfilled as part of a primary process mediated wish/phantasy, *and* whose present content will *later* serve the practice function for survival and reproductive selective fitness, will be wishes properly functioning under full Normal conditions.[27]

What I have been arguing for concerning a proper-function account for the mechanisms producing primary process mediated phantasies and wishes and for some of the phantasy and wish states produced, can best be summed up by making additions (shown by brackets) to Millikan's own (1993, p. 67) statement cited above:

> [T]*he mechanisms in us that manufacture desires* [*and those producing primary process mediated phantasies and wishes*]... have proliferated because the desires [and phantasies and wishes] they produce are sometimes relevant to our flourishing and reproducing, and because relevant desires [and primary process mediated phantasies and wishes] have sometimes participated in processes that ultimately effected their fulfillment.

Primary process phantasies and wishes are relevant to our survival and reproductive success when they are properly functioning under conditions by which they enhance selective fitness via practice for the future. Playing, by phantasizing and wishing p, where the content of p concerns vital matters, can enhance biological fitness if the three following conditions are met: (1) if phantasizing and wishing p takes place at a time t when p does not yet obtain; (2) if p does obtain at a later time, $t+1$; and (3) if, when p does obtain at $t+1$, the wishful phantasy of p at time t will have provided a practice for p, a practice which affords selective success. Insofar as these conditions for the proper functioning of primary process phantasies and wishes are the Normal conditions, it is these Normal conditions that will fix the content of these phantasies and wishes appropriately, *in the absence of rationality*.

If this proposed proper function Normal condition account for primary process mediated mechanisms for phantasy and wish (and for some of the phantasy and wish states produced) goes through successfully, Millikan's view of mental content can readily accommodate the primary processes as

---

27 In Chapter 8 another important distinction between wishes and desires will be addressed, namely that for desires, but not for wishes, there is a central role for an agent's action toward fulfillment.

a-rational, yet having mental content. And if the Millikan position can indeed so accommodate the primary processes, the attributionism objection—so serious an objection that it challenges this very conception of the primary processes—can be considered undermined and refuted.[28]

Conclusion

In this chapter I argued against the case made by mainstream attributionist philosophers that the very concept of contentful primary process a-rational mentation is incoherent. By both countering the attributionist arguments and providing a positive account for such mentation, I have taken a step toward establishing that the a-rational primary processes *can* indeed be mental and contentful. In the following part—Part IV consisting of Chapter 6 on drives; Chapter 7 on phantasies, beliefs, and neurotic beliefs; and Chapter 8 on desires—I will take the next step, making the bolder claim that the a-rational primary processes *are* mental and contentful. This claim is made because (1) in other work of an empirical nature, using convergent evidence, my colleagues and I have shown that primary processes exist (Brakel *et al.*, 2000, 2002; Brakel 2004; Brakel and Shevrin 2005); (2) in the current chapter I have made a case for the plausibility of the primary processes existing as contentful; and (3) to not do so would leave a number of psychological events seemingly unexplainable, denying what seems to be a clear casual role played by contentful primary process phantasies and wishes. In short, without the claim that a-rational primary processes exist and exist as contentful and meaningful, a rather depleted understanding of human motivation and intention remains, one based mainly on a standard psychological belief/desire analysis and allowing but a very limited philosophy of human action.

---

[28] Note, I am proposing here only *one way* for *a certain category of wishes and phantasies* to have a plausible proper function in the Millikanian sense. For other categories of wishes and phantasies, even if the play-as-practice explanation will not serve, there is no reason to rule out the possibility of a different sort of Millikanian proper function account. For example, a plausible proper function account might be advanced for certain types of primary process phantasies and wishes in terms of their contents providing material for creative thought. See Brakel (2007) for an abbreviated review of accounts of primary process reflecting creativity.

Part IV

A philosophy of action view of psychoanalysis

Following from the work in Part III / Chapter 5, Part IV concerns applications of the concept of a-rational yet contentful primary process (Corollary One) to several areas, all at the interface of psychoanalysis and the philosophy of action. Chapter 6, "Drive theory and primary process," deals with the psychoanalytic concept of drive and in particular takes up the non-singular (primary process) nature of drive-objects. Employing once again a proper function naturalistic account, I will demonstrate that a distinction can be made between the indeterminate, on the one hand, and the not singularly determinate, on the other. Further in Chapter 6, the philosophical issue of vagueness is considered in relation to the determinate-yet-not-singularly-determinate drive-objects. Here I will argue that primary process concepts, despite superficial appearances, are not vague concepts.

Chapter 7 "Phantasies, beliefs, and neurotic-beliefs" and Chapter 8 "Desires and the willingness to act," are the two most clinical chapters, and they deal most directly with the inadequacies in attempting to understand human psychology and action only in terms of conscious belief/desire analyses, that is, with neither Freud's Assumption Three—that there is contentful unconscious mentation, nor his Corollary One—that contentful a-rational primary processes exist—in place. Both Chapters 7 and 8 also present the consequences of confusions of one sort of psychological attitude for another. Chapter 7 makes the case that neurotic-beliefs, while actually having the structure of phantasies, are experienced as beliefs and treated as though they have the causal role of beliefs. Chapter 8 argues for "the readiness-to-act" as the constitutive function of desire, and highlights the troubles that ensue when desires are seen as merely unacceptable wishes.

Chapter 6

Drive theory and primary process[1]

Drives defined and described

Drive theory in psychoanalysis concerns the "instinctual drives." Currently there is much controversy regarding the relation between instinctual drives and affects. Although for some theorists these are placed in a single category, as will soon be illustrated, the very philosophical analysis I am undertaking here presupposes a fundamental difference between drives and affects. Thus, while much of the account of drives provided in this chapter concerns the objects of drives or "drive-objects," particularly the nature of the contents of drive-objects, the very notion of an "affect object" is incoherent. One cannot, for instance, consider something or someone to be the object of my depression, even in those cases in which this something or someone contributes most clearly and significantly to its cause. Further, not only are affects without contentful objects, unlike drives which always tend toward something with a directional vector, affects have no aims; they do not point. Thus, as these are substantive differences, not merely differences in usage, one can conclude that drives and affects belong to two distinct categories.

While the confounding of conceptual categories for drive and affect might be the latest problem drive theory is facing, it has not been its only one. At various times and in various quarters there have been great rhetorical debates and confusions about Freud's very use of the term "drive." For the purpose of this chapter however (because the terminological issue is not relevant to the philosophical analysis) I will use what has become "the" (or at least "a")

[1] This chapter is slightly revised from two earlier versions. It was presented as "Drive Theory and Primary Process: A Philosophical Account" at the Panel on "Psychoanalysis, Cognitive-Neuroscience and the Philosophy of Mind: Shared and Unshared Ground" for Division 39 (Psychoanalytic Division), Annual Meetings of the American Psychological Association, Miami, March 2004; and it appears under the same title in (P. Giampieri-Deutsch (ed.), *Psychoanalysis as an Empirical Interdisciplinary Science: Collected Papers on Contemporary Psychoanalytic Research*, Chapter 3, pp.75–90, Vienna: The Austrian Academy of Sciences Press, 2005.

standard reading (according to Nagera 1969, 1970) starting with Freud's (1905b) comments from *Three Essays on Sexuality*:

> By an "instinct" [henceforth to be translated as "instinctual drive" or just "drive"] is provisionally to be understood [as] the psychical representative of an endosomatic ... source of stimulation ... the concept of instinctual drive is thus one of those lying on the frontier between the mental and the physical. The simplest and likeliest assumption ... would seem to be that in itself an instinctual drive is without quality, and, so far as the mental life is concerned, only to be regarded as a measure of the demand made upon the mind for work. What distinguishes the instinctual drives from one another and endows them with specific qualities is their relation to their somatic sources and to their aims. (p. 168)

In *Instincts and Their Vicissitudes*, Freud (1915a), after using almost identical words to define the instinctual drives, elaborated four terms needed for fully characterizing the concept. In addition to the "source" and "aims" of an instinctual drive, described in the earlier work, he added the "pressure" of a drive and its "object." (pp. 122–3):

> By the *pressure* [my italics] of an instinctual drive we understand its motor factor, the amount of force or the measure of the demand for work which it represents ...
> ... The *aim* [my italics] of an instinctual drive is in every instance satisfaction ... obtained by removing the state of stimulation at the source of the instinctual drive. But although the ultimate aim of each instinctual drive remains unchangeable, there may yet be different paths leading to the same ultimate aim; so that an instinctual drive may be found to have various nearer or intermediate aims ...
> ... The *object* [my italics] of an instinctual drive is the thing ... through which the instinctual drive is able to achieve its aim. It is what is most variable about an instinctual drive and is not originally connected with it, but becomes assigned to it only in consequence of being peculiarly fitted to make satisfaction possible. The object is not necessarily extraneous; it may equally well be a part of the subject's own body. It may be changed any number of times in the course of the vicissitudes which the instinctual drive undergoes ....It may happen that the same object serves for the satisfaction of several instinctual drives simultaneously ...
> ... By the *source* [my italics] of an instinctual drive is meant the somatic process which occurs in an organ or part of the body and whose stimulus is represented in mental life by an instinctual drive.

In sum then, an instinctual drive is the mental representative of a physiologic need state such that a certain pressure or quantitative demand for work, having a certain quality varying with particular drives, is placed on the psychological apparatus toward fulfillment and thereby cessation of the particular instinctual drive. Each instinctual drive in addition to its pressure, has a source (in the body), an aim (the distal part of which is always fulfillment, the proximal part varies with each type of instinctual drive and is the mode to achieve fulfillment), and an object. The object is that thing or those things or parts of things (which can include the self, and other beings) through which satisfaction can be obtained. The source, aim, and object of an instinctual drive determine its qualitative nature. The pressure of a drive, mostly originating from its somatic source, constitutes the quantitative contribution.

An example: X's oral drives

X is an eight-month-old baby, and X is hungry. X has a number of oral instinctual drives—to suck, to swallow, and to feel the pleasure associated with pleasant tastes and temperatures and the comfort of gradual gastric fullness replacing emptiness. The somatic *sources* are falling blood sugar, hypothalamic regulation and signaling, gastric stirrings, and a certain set of sensations in the mouth. The *aims* are, distally to have this drive state reduced, and proximally to get fed. The *objects* are whatever will satisfy these oral instinctual drives. Food, not separable from whomever or whatever (in part or whole) provides it, is an obvious object; but so are the pacifier, the rattle, and part of the blanket— whatever is good to suck on. Thus for Baby X the objects of these oral drives are X's mother's left breast and nipple and her right breast and nipple, and a bottle and nipple, and X's father's face as he holds X and the bottle, and the milk, and mother's face, and how it feels being held and fed, and how these faces and breasts (and bottles) look, and the pacifier and the hand of its provider, and the blanket edge, especially how it feels in X's mouth—any part of this and all of it together.

A philosophical account of drives

Drives and propositional-attitude psychology

Instinctual drives do not fit well into the propositional-attitude psychology favored by many philosophers (including the attributionists discussed in Chapter 5) to account for motivation, intention, and behavior. The propositional-attitude psychology of such philosophers (1) assumes that persons having propositional attitudes are largely rational and therefore interpretable, and (2) employs contents of a particular pair of propositional attitudes—belief and desire—to understand motivation, intention, and behavior. In fact, belief/desire psychology and the more general term propositional-attitude psychology are often used synonymously.

Belief is a type of cognitive propositional attitude—cognitive, as in having to do with knowledge and perception. Supposition and hypothesis are other cognitive attitudes. Desire is a type of conative propositional attitude—conative pertaining to striving and volition. Wish and drive are other conative propositional attitudes. Desires, especially when paired with beliefs, fit readily into the propositional-attitude scheme. A typical belief/desire analysis looks like this: Ms B is heading toward the Michigan Theatre now. Why? Because, as she told me earlier today, she wants (desires) to see the movie Spiderman; and because she believes it will be playing at the Michigan Theatre in ten minutes.

But do drives fit as well in propositional-attitude psychology explanations? I maintain they do not. Therefore several questions arise, the most immediate being, on what grounds do I make this assertion? Then, if I am right, why is it that drives do not allow the same sort of propositional attitude analysis? Finally, relatedly and perhaps most vitally, what is the essential difference between drives and desires that makes this the case?

Before I attend to these questions, it must be noted that there are some ways in which drives can and do admit of a standard propositional-attitude analysis. Both drives and desires can be used in conjunction with behavior to infer the content of various cognitive propositional attitudes. For example, if Mr A says he desires a cool drink, and ten seconds later is seen walking toward a water-fountain and then bending to drink, one can infer that he *believes* that water-fountains are sources of cool drinks, and further that this particular water-fountain is operational. Similarly, if we know the state of Mr A's drives, and observe certain actions he performs, the very same belief contents (and in addition the contents of his desire) can be inferred, even without any report from Mr A. Suppose, for example, it is learned that Mr A has been deprived of fluids for some time. This state will, assuming Mr A is normal, lead to heightening of the various oral instinctual drives pertaining to thirst. If in this condition he is seen approaching a water-fountain, his beliefs about water-fountains in general and this water-fountain in particular, and his desire for a drink can all be readily inferred. Conversely, drives, like desires, can themselves often be inferred given various cognitive propositional attitudes. Mr A's starting to drink from a water-fountain usually implies that he believes that water-fountains are sources for cold water, and that the particular water-fountain he is about to drink from works. From here it can be inferred not only that he is drinking because he desires a drink, but also that he does so in part owing to the various oral instinctual drives active when he is thirsty. Now of course this sort of belief/desire/drive propositional attitude analysis can go wrong. Mr A could be a water-fountain inspector, with oral drives that are well satisfied, no desire whatever for cool drinks, and a belief that the water-fountain in question is in need of repair. But most of the time the sort of propositional-attitude analysis performed on Mr A will go through, even when dealing with drives.

So why am I suggesting that instinctual drives do not fit the standard propositional-attitude psychology account? How are drives different? The answers begins with recognizing that whereas with any desire (or belief) its object can be picked out by a mental representation the content of which is singularly determinate, no such uniquely determinate content will do for the object of a drive. The representations of the objects of drives in fact look radically indeterminate in content. (See Velleman 2002, p. 90.) Mr A's desire for a cool drink has as its object "cool drink" and he has a mental representation of this. Whatever the nature of mental representations, Mr A's mental representation of cool drink, refers singularly to cool drinks. Turning now to the object of Mr A's oral drives—those fueling his desire for a cool drink, which include strivings to relieve both local mouth dryness and to increase hydration in response to more generalized signals—there is no such straightforward analysis. The object of these drives, hence the content of the mental representation picking out the object, cannot be specified as singular and determinate, anymore in Mr A's case than for Baby X above. The object can be approximated as some sort of set and/ or amalgam of objects and parts of objects, all and whatever of which will bring forth a satisfied feeling in Mr A's mouth and a relieved feeling overall. But any mental representation of this sort of drive-object will seem "either radically inde-terminate in content or … [to be] playing a non-standard role" (Velleman 2002, p. 90). Velleman (2002 p. 91) describes such representations as "far too vague to be expressed in the concepts with which we consciously reason." He, in discussing the object of aggressive drives, continues (p. 91):

> If … we insist on framing a written or spoken "that" clause to express the content of aggression, we shall have to concede that what the [aggressive drive] attitude can … be satisfied by … [is] not only the literal truth of the clause but also indefinitely many other outcomes related only by analogy, by metaphorical similarity, or by other mental associations of an open-ended variety.

Velleman concludes (2002, p. 91), "Either way, propositional-attitude psychology will not afford the same computational advantages in this case as it does in the case of ordinary beliefs and desires, whose tendencies … to be satisfied can be summed up in sentences of ordinary language."

Thus, insofar as philosophers of mind hold that no true mental state can be radically indeterminate, and since the usual propositional-attitude determina-tion will not work for determining the objects of drives, we are left with the question—just how can the objects of drives be established as contentful? I will return to this vexing problem after a brief foray into an easier one, which follows just below.

Are drive aims singular and determinate?

That instinctual drives have objects that cannot be represented in a univocal, determinate way is central to drives not admitting of a standard propositional-attitude psychology analysis. But is the same absence of singular determinancy true of the content of drive aims? In Freud's (1915a, p. 122) basic definitions, it is clear that the aim of any drive will consist of two parts: the "ultimate and unchangeable" aim of having the state of stimulation cease through discharge and satisfaction, and the "different paths" such that a drive may have "various nearer or intermediate aims." Given this compound aim for any drive, the contents of the nearer/intermediate aims of a drive certainly seem under the threat of indeterminancy. Indeed Anna Freud (1936) in her classic work on the ego defenses, describes the aims of drives as easily modified, transformed, and displaced one for another. In a later work she (1981) states: "An individual who finds the path to an instinctual [drive] aim of adulthood blocked by internal or external obstacles can respond to such a frustration by reverting to childhood forms of satisfaction" (p. 248). And she notes that this can go in the opposite direction too: "under the influence of the superego, primitive [drive] impulses are transformed, inhibited in their aims, and the drive energies belonging to them deflected to moral, ethical, or socially higher aims" (p. 247). All of Freud's cases too (see especially Dora in Freud 1905a; Little Hans in Freud 1909; The Rat Man in Freud 1909; and The Wolf Man in Freud 1918) show abundant evidence of displaced aims. Moreover from a theoretical viewpoint, Freud seems quite convinced that drive aims were neither singular nor fixed. Despite many revisions over the years in his conceptions of regression, symptom formation, and sublimation, one thing is left unchanged: regression, symptom formation, and sublimation each remained dependent on what for Freud was obvious—that the aims of drives could be readily displaced. (See Freud 1900, 1915a, 1915b, 1926, 1940.)

Yet, although the foregoing may suggest indeterminacy of drive aims, in fact, the very nature of the transformability or displace-ability of the aims of drives, depends on one aspect being determinately fixed. Drives each have *original aims*, represented in a singular fixed fashion, and it is *from these original aims* that there can be displacement. There is support for this understanding from Freud (1905b, p. 168) in his *Three Essays on Sexuality*. "What distinguishes the instinctual drives one from another and endows them with specific qualities is their relation to their somatic sources and to their [particular] aims." Discussing Freud's allusion to the "nearer and intermediate aims" Rapaport (1957, p. 831) comments: "Freud used the term 'aim' in two different senses. One of these is the tendency toward discharge; the other … is not the universal discharge tendency itself, but something more specific." The more specific quality of an aim is determined by the "instinctual mode,"[2] each mode associated with the

---

[2] According to Rapaport (1957, p. 832), "instinctual mode" is a concept originated by Erikson (1950).

source of an instinctual drive. (p. 832). Thus as a child gaining anal sphincter control is in the anal phase, the anal drives are associated with original aims whose mode concerns retaining and expelling. Anal phase drives of course far outlast the anal phase of development. Drives with aims to *retain* household junk, for example, or to *expel* anger are commonplace; but no more so than are *displacements from these original anal phase aims*. For example, the aim to retain can be displaced onto the perhaps more socially acceptable aim of collecting works of art; while the aim to expel can be displaced onto creating such works. Thus with respect to the proximal aims, particular instinctual modes each have their own original aims. These have fixed univocal content, and it is *from these original aims* that displacements take place.

Drive-objects are not singular. Must they be indeterminate?

The threat of indeterminancy for the content of drive-objects cannot be removed so easily. While the case has been made for drives having original singular and determinate aims from which displacements occur, there is not a parallel case for drive-objects. Returning to Freud's (1915a, 122–3) definition of instinctual drive-object, he states: "It is what is most variable about an instinct[ual drive] and is *not originally* connected with it, but becomes assigned to it only in consequence of being peculiarly fitted to make satisfaction possible." With drives possessing no specified original objects through which to gain discharge and satisfaction, the role of drive-object can be filled by any person, material object, part or combination thereof, fitting a drive in order to make satisfaction possible; and any person, material object, part or combination thereof is as good as any other.

Velleman (2002, p. 90), in discussing his own aggressive drive gives a convincing description of the non-singularity of drive-objects. While performing various kicks in Tae Kwon Do exercises, he found that his "aggression could be turned on virtually any solid object, including any person who happened to be my assigned opponent."

Rapaport (1960) also recognized the non-singularity of drive-objects. He makes the claim that the assignment of object to drive in consequence of good fit for gratification implied "a coordination of the instinctual drive discharge with a *definite (even if broad) range of objects* [my emphasis], and an equifinality in regard to this range of objects" (p. 878).[3] Rapaport (p. 878) further held that what constitutes the range of well-fitted objects was likely "phylogenetically determined." Earlier (1957, p. 833) he noted a parallel between

---

[3] Note that Rapaport's assertion that the range is "definite" will not suffice to ensure determinancy.

Freud's set of drive-objects and the "releasers" in Lorenz's system of innate releasing mechanisms (the most well known of which is imprinting), reporting that Lorenz (1950) and Timbergen (1951) found that the releasers were not singular objects. Rather that they were "aggregates of stimuli, only some of which are indispensable for effecting adequate release, and various combinations of which can effect adequate release." (The quotation is from Rapaport, 1957, p. 833.)

This finding accords remarkably well with the above description of the object of Baby X's oral drive. This object was said to be the set which includes any amalgam or part of the provider of satisfaction and/or the material object satisfying Baby X's oral drive: X's mother's left breast and nipple and her right breast and nipple and a bottle and nipple, and father's face as he holds the bottle, and the milk, and how it feels being held and fed, and how X's mother's face and breast look, and the pacifier and the hand of its provider, and the blanket edge, especially how it feels in X's mouth—any part of this and all of it together.

Two things can be seen in these examples of drive-objects: (1) There is no primacy or originality of one part of these objects over another. In other words, displacement from some original drive-object is not taking place here as it does for drive aims. (2) These objects do not appear singular and determinate, at least not in any ordinary way. Instead, the objects of drives are either parts or amalgams of persons or items—as is seen in the Baby X oral object example and with the animals studied by Lorenz and Timbergen—or drive-objects consist of a set of items linked by some contingent inessential feature—as is the case in Velleman's example of "any solid object" which happened to be available.

How can these mysterious drive-objects be better understood? I do have a proposal, and it follows forthwith. Although drive-objects are not singularly determinate, they are not haphazard, indeterminate assortments. Objects of specific drives in fact can be described as category members belonging to distinct categories predicated on more than just the trivial (but essential) fact that all such members must be drive-gratifying. The discrete coherent categories to which drive-objects belong are all of a particular nature. They *are a-rational primary process categories* whose members are grouped together, not at all randomly, but lawfully, albeit not according to secondary process rational principles. Instead, primary process categories cohere and are organized according to the several associative, a-rational principles of the primary processes. (See Freud 1900, 1915b, 1926, 1940 for various statements of these principles and Chapters 4 and 5.) There is one type of primary process category, for example, in which category membership is determined on the basis of a shared feature, one that is not an essential attribute[4]—but instead is the sort of feature occasioning the associative linking often seen in the primary process dominated content of manifest dreams and free associations. Illustrative of drive-object categories constituted in this way are (1) Lorenz's ducklings, imprinting onto any moving item of a certain physical size, (2) Velleman, who would kick any solid object, and (3) Baby X, who sucks on anything that has in common only a shape that can fit in a baby's mouth. Another primary process associative principle links and/or makes an amalgam of elements that are spatially contiguous. Primary process drive-object categories can form in this way too, namely, Baby X's oral drive-objects which include not only mother's left nipple and the milk which flows from it, but also father's hand, contiguous to the bottle of milk that he holds, and the face of a parent, adjacent to the vessel with milk, and so forth.[5]

But even given drive-objects that can be well described in terms of particular primary process categories, we still have a problem: Can primary process objects be represented, and if so, how?

Can primary process objects be represented? How?

The work of the last section demonstrated that drive-objects can be better understood when they are seen as collections of items and part-items that cohere on the basis of primary process principles. And yet the problem of indeterminancy still threatens because we must ask how such drive-objects, organized in primary process category form, can be represented. Given that the standard propositional-attitude psychology analyses used for individuating representations of the singular objects of desires or beliefs will not work—and they will not work precisely because drives are not standard propositional attitudes with singular, representable objects—is there some analysis that can fix the content of these objects of drives?

---

[4] There is an *essential* aspect joining all members of what I have termed a drive-object category. All members must be capable of satisfying the drive (at least to some extent). The *inessential* aspect is in respect to the various members themselves. Thus, persons, pieces of furniture, and rocks are related as "solid objects one could kick," but solid-such-that-it-is-suitable-for-kicking is not an essential feature of rocks, furniture, or persons. Likewise members of the category "things that babies can suck upon" *essentially*, from the perspective of a drive-object, must be things, parts or wholes of which can be put in babies' mouths. But these are *inessential* features of the great majority of items that babies do put in their mouths.

[5] The topic of primary process categorizations has been addressed much more fully in Brakel (2002, 2003, 2004) in Brakel *et al.* (2000, 2002), and Brakel and Shevrin (2005).

Again, any of the usual type of content fixing must be ruled out at the onset—like that employed by the attributionists[6]—wherein interpretability follows from rationality that is assumed normatively. How could this work when we are dealing with a-rational, albeit lawfully organized content? What would work as an account with different normative assumptions, yet an account not susceptible to the indeterminancy problem? These requirements can be met using the proper-function naturalism developed by Ruth Millikan (1984, 1993). Here the normative assumptions of selective fitness success and evolutionary explanation replace those of interpretative success and rational explanation.

In the sections that follow I will briefly describe fitness-based normativity and proper-function explanations, showing how they can be used to fix both the contents of beliefs and the contents of a rather more unusual type of cognitive process. Then in keeping with this analysis, I will claim that primary process based drive-objects too can have fixed, yet determinate non-singular contents insofar as these primary process organized drive-objects indeed have a proper-function, one which under certain conditions can lead to fitness success.[7]

Fitness based proper-function and the contents of beliefs

First, to demonstrate selective fitness normativity, let us start with something simple and far afield—sweat glands (see Millikan 1993, pp. 73–4.). The function of sweat glands is to secrete sweat. But their "proper-function" entails what Millikan (1993) terms Normal conditions. Normal conditions are those in which properly functioning sweat glands contributed to the survival of animals possessing them and thereby increased the selective success of those animals. Thus, when there is a tumor pressing on the temperature-sensing center, sweat glands funtioning flawlessly and producing sweat with the body at its regular temperature, are not performing their Normal proper-function, because they are not functioning under Normal conditions. Only those sweat glands producing sweat when the body is overheated are sweat glands properly functioning under Normal conditions, that is, conditions contributing to the animal's selective reproductive advantage.

---

[6] For attributionist and other rationality based views, see especially Davidson, 1980, 1984; Cherniak, 1981; Stich, 1983; and Dennett, 1978, 1987; and for a brief summary of these views see Chapter 5 above.)

[7] What follows is an application to drive-object contents of the argument appearing in Chapter 5 (and in Brakel 2002). In the interest of clarity I must rehearse the background for the original argument. I apologize for the redundancy to those who have read Chapter 5.

Now, let us apply this to an area of much more moment for this project, beliefs. Specifically we are concerned with how the object of a belief—what a belief is about, that is, its content—gets singularly and determinately represented. Not all beliefs are properly-functioning under Normal conditions. The Normal/selective fitness conferring conditions were those in which the truth conditions of the belief's content (i.e. the object of belief as represented) matched the truth conditions obtaining in the world. In other words, only true beliefs are those properly-functioning under Normal conditions (Millikan 1993, p. 73). But note that in Millikan's program there is nothing *a priori* or necessary in the contents of beliefs matching truth conditions in the world, or in believers coming by the objects of their beliefs rationally. Rather, true beliefs and the rationality they usually entail, are contingently determined biological norms. Yes, it happens to have been the case that our ancestors capable of rationally mediated true beliefs, and exercising this capacity frequently enough, had selective advantages such that the mechanisms supporting true-belief generation were reproduced. But that the Normal conditions for beliefs are those in which the truth conditions for the content represented are constituted by the truth conditions of the world is entirely a contingent matter. Note also that the Normal conditions need not be the typical conditions. Provided that there are enough Normal properly-functioning beliefs to fix content via fitness success and selective normativity, instances of abNormally functioning beliefs, that is, false beliefs, incomplete beliefs, and so on will also have content.

A proper-function account of toad representation

Also related to our interest in fixing content for primary process drive-objects, let us examine how the objects of toad perceptual representations are fixed using a proper-function Normal condition account. Toad perception is instructive as it can be used to demonstrate (1) representational content without any rationality, (2) abNormal instances that are nonetheless contentful, and (3) representations that have fixed determinate content despite initial appearances to the contrary. Toads, Millikan (1993, p. 109) claims, have contentful representations of bugs, despite their incapacity to distinguish bugs from lead pellets. Toads have a powerful set of reflexes such that when bugs *or* lead pellets are within striking distance, tongue protrusion, item capture, and item swallowing ensue in rapid sequence. Lots of bugs and lots of pellets are swallowed indiscriminately; and yet Millikan claims that toads have a determinate representation of bugs. Here is how: Although a toad cannot differentiate a bug from a lead pellet, presumably producing indistinguishable visual representations, only those representations of actual bugs are the result of properly-functioning Normal condition representations.

Why? Because, it is the case that only actual bugs have contributed to toad nutrition and thereby to toad reproductive success. And what about those representations deriving from actual lead pellets? They are not properly-functioning Normal condition representations of bugs. Nor are they any sort of representations of lead pellets. They are abNormal representation of bugs! The content "bug" is fixed in a determinate fashion according to selective fitness normativity.

A proper-function account of primary process drive-objects

Finally, we can take up a proper-function selective fitness argument for fixing content in primary process drive-objects. A proper-function account is given in two steps. The initial step is to list the criteria for "proper-function"; remembering that proper-functioning must be functioning that is both without flaw or defect *and* occurring under conditions that would enhance selective fitness, the so-called Normal conditions. The second step is to propose the Normal or fitness enhancing conditions.

Step One: Three criteria for proper-function for primary process drive-objects

First, for a proper-function account of primary process drive-objects it must be established that the drive-objects in question are indeed linked by a primary process principle constituting a primary process organized category. In other words, the members or elements comprising the objects of a drive must be connected in a primary process fashion—not in a random way. They must cohere in accord with primary process principles, which include association by the similarity of inessential features, and/or condensation (amalgamation) and displacement (associative linking) operating on elements contiguous in time and/or space.

Second, any proper-function account of drive-objects necessitates that the objects in question satisfy the drive aims—both the proximal aims specific to particular drives, and the ultimate aim of drive discharge.

A final and most important criterion for the proper-function account of primary process organized drive-objects is as follows. It must be the case that it is the very diversity and variability, the non-singularity, of the drive-objects as constituted by their primary process nature that contributes to sufficient drive satisfaction.[8]

---

[8] Rapaport (1957, p. 833) alludes to this third criterion being the case: "The coordination of instinctual drive and object is assumed to be innate, that is, given by evolution ... it is relatively flexible ... [with] variability in the object of the instinctual drive."

Step Two: Normal conditions for primary process drive-objects

Having specified the proper-function for primary process drive-objects, the next step is to propose those conditions under which the proper-functioning of these drive-objects would lead to selective reproductive fitness success. If found, these will be the Normal conditions—the conditions that allow the primary process drive-objects to have fixed determinate content, without being univocal and singular. This is a surprisingly easy task, because here the Normal conditions are the typical and usual conditions.

Let us look at the consequences if primary process groupings of objects did *not* comprise drive-objects. Suppose Lorenz's ducklings could only imprint uniquely onto their mothers. Yes, if you are a duckling it is ideal to imprint onto your mother; but suppose she is gone or sick? Isn't better to be able to imprint onto some other conspecifics (or even onto a researcher) and have a chance thereby to survive and reproduce? There seems to be clear selective fitness advantage in the diversity of the primary process organized "releasers" ducklings possess.

Similarly, with human babies, if Baby X's oral drives could only be quelled with mother's milk from her nipples, Baby X would likely be hungry most of the time, certainly discontent much of the time, and plausibly less likely to grow up healthy enough to reproduce.

Now jumping ahead developmentally, suppose drives from the Oedipal phase could have but a unique, singular type of object. Wouldn't Oedipal phase resolution be even harder than it is? Wouldn't choices for mates be severely curtailed, at the detriment to both individual and species?

If we turn to aggression, the same potential benefit for primary process objects vs. a unique singular object can be seen. Suppose for some people the "aggressive drive" had as its object only conspecifics, those vying for a mate, or those attacking first, and so on. These people would be at a selective disadvantage with respect to nourishment compared with those whose aggressive drive also included prey and predator animals. The fitness disadvantage would be no less for people whose aggressive drive had the singular object of big predators. These people would have trouble defending themselves and progeny against attacks from other people, as well as from noxious, but small animals (such as snakes and spiders). They might also be at a calorie disadvantage, finding less aggressive drive pleasure in fishing and small game hunting.

Thus, with these two steps I have made a case for a proper-function account of primary process constituted drive-objects. First, that there are criteria for the proper-function of primary process based drive-objects—namely, that the members comprising the drive-objects are not singularly determinate but instead are categories constituted according to primary process principles; and that it is owing to this very diversity generated by their primary process organization that the resultant drive-objects yield adequate drive satisfaction. Second, that there are Normal conditions under which the diversity facilitated by the primary process drive-objects *can* enhance fitness success. Hence, the argument goes through: these primary process drive-objects can have content that is both non-singular and yet determinate, with selective fitness normativity underwriting the constraint against indeterminacy.

Psychoanalytic concluding remarks: Transference

Transferences are manifestations of primary process organized drive-objects. Since I feel XYZ about Person Q and you resemble him with respect to superficial characteristic *c*, I feel XYZ about you. Transferences are ubiquitous. Since drives never cease, arising continually and requiring satisfaction; and primary process connections for drive-objects, while not unconstrained, have no numerical limit—it is hardly surprising that quickly formed, but sometimes deep transferences occasioned by superficial resemblances are not unusual in any setting; and that intense transferences in psychoanalyses—facilitated by the intimacy and quiet of the analytic situation, which allow drive pressures of all sorts to come to the fore—are almost inevitable.

The philosophical analysis offered in this chapter takes as given entities such as these transferences, where drive-objects organized in a primary process fashion are evident to psychoanalysts. From here a serious philosophical problem—the threat of indeterminate content for drive-objects—was raised and resolved. If there is a distinctly new psychoanalytic issue brought to light by this philosophical analysis, it is whether we should continue to view transferences as displacements from some "original" object or whether with respect to drive-objects, the whole notion of "singularly original" must be reconsidered.

Philosophical concluding remarks: Vague concepts, the mental content of toads, and primary process drive-objects

What is the relation of the representations/contents of primary process drive-objects, to those representations toads have regarding bugs and lead pellets, and to those contents or representations associated with "vague concepts," an important topic in philosophy? Williamson (1994) in his tour de force book, *Vagueness*, after an exhaustive review of all competing positions, essentially favors the "epistemic view," on which vague concepts result from our human cognitive limitations.

The epistemic view hinges on the idea that "knowledge involving vague concepts [is] a distinct species of the genus, inexact knowledge" (Williamson 1994, p. 217).

Just as there *is* a precise number marking the quantity of hairs on my head, but this is a specific number I certainly do not now know, vague concepts—such as crowd, heap, thin, old—likewise *are* (or at least could be) picking out something precise ontologically that I (and other humans) just do not know. Thus, on this view, there *is* one and only one number that represents the precise number of people gathered (in a particular situation) such that they will now constitute a crowd, and there *is* a particular number of grains in this specific sand pile such that it first constitutes a heap. The problem is that our human concepts "heap" and "crowd" are vague. Likewise take borderline cases of rather ordinary concepts used as descriptors like, thin, bald, old. Again on the epistemic view, there *is* a fact of the matter whether or not some specific X is thin, Y is bald, and Z is old, and so on—however our cognitive limitations, do not let *us* know the cut-off points as to what constitutes thin vs. not-thin, bald vs. not-bald, old vs. not-old in each specific case.

The notion of vague concepts becomes easier to understand when we look at toads' representations of bugs and lead pellets. From the human perspective, toads' concept of bug is vague. Toads cannot distinguish bugs from lead pellets, and presumably represent them identically. Although this representation, on the proper-function view I have been propounding, always refers to bugs—correctly when there is a bug to ingest, and incorrectly when a lead pellet is swallowed—there *is* a correct representation, one that we can know, but toads cannot. So although toads' representations are good enough, if toads were better cognizers then they too would be able to make the distinction between bugs and lead pellets. And if this were the case, perhaps there would be some selective advantage—fewer ingestings of non-nutritive items, which even if not harmful take up the time and space that could be devoted to real bugs.

Representations of primary process organized drive-objects may seem analogous to vague concepts too; epistemologically no singular object for drives can be discerned. But I will argue (1) that this analogy can be only superficial because the *ontology* of a particular drive-object, unlike that of the number of grains in that particular heap, *is not in fact singular*; and (2) that any notion of a deep analogy rests on an insufficient understanding of the nature of the primary process mental content in general, and the nature of primary process drive-objects in particular.

Regarding primary process content itself, consider that *intrinsically* this content might be neither vague nor indeterminate; but only seem so *relative* to the secondary process terms in which we (as secondary process dominated thinkers) are forced to formulate it. (See Chapter 4.) Perhaps for any representational system (and this would have to include that of the toads and their bugs/lead pellets) there is in itself, from within it, no vagueness or indeterminacy, but only the appearance of such when there is an attempt to translate it into a *relatively* more precise and determinate representational system. While the more precise and determinate second system is capable of the distinctions that the first system cannot make, the formulation or translation may not be workable, a situation which does not imply the vagueness or indeterminacy of the first system content.[9,10]

Let us turn now to the nature of primary process drive-objects. Indeed, as I look at the crowd at University of Michigan football stadium, it seems equally likely that there are 99,546 people as 99,000 people as 98,765 people. The set of numbers comprising my representation of the count of people making up this crowd is vague; and so is the set of numbers I offer when asked at which point the group of people become constituted as a crowd.[11] In both cases the sets of numbers representing my guesses are vague; and the elements I single out when I do give numbers are arbitrary and random. While it may seem to be that a similarly unconstrained string of random and arbitrary elements comprise primary process drive-objects, this is not the case. First, and most fundamentally, the multiple member drive-object category must be derived according to its proper-function, following primary process organizational principles toward a diversity that allows satisfaction. And second, at least with respect to human beings, each drive-object category is further constrained by the need for each of its constituent elements to be subjectively (if idiosyncratically) and specifically relevant to the particular person (or animal) with the drive. Thus *my* mother's face will not suffice to satisfy the oral drives of Baby X; and the realm of possible Oedipal choices for me will not be the same as the realm for you.

Further, while without human cognitive limitations one could more correctly know the number of people at the U of M stadium, improving cognitive capabilities could not increase one's ability to constitute a "more correct" drive-object, as drive fulfillment does not admit of "correct" or "incorrect." And yet one could wonder, would fewer cognitive limitations allow "better" (if not more correct) drive-objects, objects that fitted better the environment,

---

[9] The difficulty dreamers have in adequately describing particular dreams can be explained on this basis. The translation/transformation from the primary process manifest dream to the secondary process mediated remembering and recounting can only be but partly successful. (See Chapter 4, p. 56)

[10] I thank David Velleman for help in working out the ideas in this paragraph.

[11] These examples might illustrate nicely the relationship Williamson wants to draw between inexact knowledge (the actual number of people in the U of M stadium) and vague concepts (what number constitutes a crowd).

toward greater satisfaction and ultimately enhanced fitness success? It is tempting to answer, yes. But at the same time it is hard to imagine any rational matching process being as resiliently successful in providing fit between drives and their objects as are the a-rational primary process drive-object categories with their built in diversity.

General conclusions

Instinctual drives, unlike desires and beliefs do not have objects with singularly determinate content. While the contents of drive-objects are fixed and not indeterminate, because they lack univocal determinacy they will not admit of the usual belief/desire standard account. Propositional attitude psychology dominated by the analysis of beliefs and desires is thus limited in its ability to explain and account for important types of human intention, and motivation. Drives and the a-rational primary process contents of drive-objects are central to human actions; so are the (often) primary process organized contents of wishes, phantasies, and another type of propositional attitude—neurotic beliefs, which will be the subject of the Chapter 7. In Chapter 7, "Phantasies, neurotic-beliefs, and beliefs-proper," it will become apparent, in fact, that only a small proportion of our actions can be properly classified as having largely conscious and rational secondary process mediated intentions and motivations— our illusions and desires[12] to the contrary notwithstanding.

---

[12] I do mean "desires" and not "wishes" here. People desire that their motivations and intentions are conscious and rational. As we will see in the Chapter 7, owing to this desire (as well as the need secondary process thinkers have to believe that they know, discussed in Chapter 4), people convince themselves of the rationality of content that is quite irrational. That they desire such, rather than merely wish it, is suggested by the fact that people actually *act* to make their intentions seem rational to themselves. This presupposes something that I will not argue for until Chapter 8, "Desire and the readiness to act," namely that the readiness to act is the constitutive function of desires, but not of wishes.

Chapter 7

Phantasies, neurotic-beliefs, and beliefs-proper[1]

Introduction

Beliefs, according to most philosophers of mind, are cognitive states that take the form of propositional attitudes. But there are three distinct types of propositional attitude, all usually considered "beliefs" that can be recognized. Beliefs of the first type, henceforth to be called "beliefs-proper" are cognitive attitudes described by philosophers as reality-tested, truth-directed, and regulated by their truth conditions insofar as beliefs-proper are held or dropped as a function of reality-tested evidence in the world for or against the belief. A belief-proper can be false and thereby believed falsely; however once probative evidence that it is false is gained, it can no longer be believed. For example, I can have a belief-proper that it is raining outside, gaining my evidence from seeing drops of water hit against my window. But what if it is not really raining and that the source of the water is from a nearby sprinkler? Then I will have a false belief-proper that it is raining. Suppose a few minutes later I go over to the window and see the sprinkler that is the source of the water drops. I can no longer believe that it is raining; further reality-tested evidence counts against this belief.

The second type of belief, "religious or social beliefs," cannot be reality-tested. As there can never be sufficient evidence accrued to know whether this sort of belief is true or false, one can hold it indefinitely, choose to relinquish it, or change it, without one's rationality being called into question. Many widely held ethical, and cultural, as well as popular and everyday beliefs belong to this category of religious or social belief. The belief that God exists is an example at one end of this spectrum, and the belief that thank-you notes should be sent by regular mail and not e-mail is an example at the other. The religious or social type of belief is not the subject of this chapter and little more will be said about it.

---

[1] This chapter is a revised version of Brakel (2001).

I am advancing "neurotic-belief" as a third type of belief. Although the phenomena to be described are well known and of great interest to psychoanalysts,
they have not been known as "neurotic-beliefs" per se. Hence I introduce the
term "neurotic-belief" as an original concept. For psychoanalytic theory, these
neurotic-beliefs are important in that they consist, as conceptualized, in meaningful dynamic unconscious contents (Assumption Three) organized in a
primary process fashion (Corollary One). Clinically they are significant too.
Often fixed and central in our neurotic patients, these neurotic-beliefs are
more like phantasies (of considerable complexity with conscious and unconscious aspects) than they are like beliefs-proper. Both phantasies and neurotic-
beliefs are propositional attitudes that can be characterized as primary process
in organization, having content that is not regulated by truth considerations,
and not subject to reality-testing. And yet because secondary process thinkers
routinely reorganize everything according to secondary process principles,[2]
not only do neurotic beliefs have a secondary process veneer, but spurious
psychic-reality[3]-based "evidence" is employed to maintain neurotic-beliefs—
evidence (mis)taken to be accrued by the reality-testing mechanisms underlying beliefs-proper. Thus, neurotic-beliefs are experienced and treated as if they
met the criteria for beliefs-proper. This has deleterious consequences, especially owing to a related characteristic of neurotic-beliefs: unlike beliefs-proper,
neurotic-beliefs with their psychic-reality foundation remain impervious to
real-world evidence. Thus, whereas new falsifying information must, and
readily does, cause one to give up false beliefs-proper, neurotic-beliefs
continue to be held nonetheless, as the holders of neurotic-beliefs tend to
discount and dismiss any contrary real-world evidence.

This state of affairs helps explain why cognitive behavioral therapies, based
on righting false beliefs, can prove disappointing. Cognitive behavioral therapies are quite effective in straightening out false beliefs-proper, but they are
ineffective when the problematic propositional attitude is not a belief-proper
at all, but a neurotic-belief. Similarly, the prevalence of neurotic-beliefs also
helps explain why the standard philosophical belief/desire propositional
attitude accounts of human psychology cannot be adequate. If in such

---

[2] For more on this tendency toward secondary process reorganization see Chapter 4, and
Chapter 6—specifically, the section "Philosophical conclusions," and below.

[3] "Psychic-reality" is a term easily understood using almost any clinical example. Three will
follow just below. But here is a working definition from *Psychoanalytic Terms and Concepts*,
edited by Moore and Fine (1990, p. 163): "*psychic-reality* designates the individual's total
subjective experiential world including thoughts, feelings, fantasies, as well as perceptions
of the external world, regardless of whether they reflect the external world."

formulations neurotic-beliefs are placed in the role of beliefs-proper, serious category errors result. Symptomatic behaviors, and other non-rational phenomena, understood only in the terms of such analyses, get characterized as somehow rational, while a real comprehension of neurotic-belief driven a-rational/irrational behaviors will prove elusive, beyond the scope of belief/desire analysis. If on the other hand belief/desire analyses are restricted to beliefs-proper, much salient and interesting human behavior, including but not restricted to the psychopathological, will be excluded.

A serious effort to classify propositional attitudes like phantasies, beliefs-proper, and neurotic-beliefs—a main goal of this chapter—can afford psychoanalysts certain advantages. By clearly defining and classifying some of these concepts central to clinical psychoanalytic phenomena, and in particular by investigating how the primary process organized states of phantasy and neurotic-belief differ from beliefs-proper, a method of analysis borrowed from philosophy can enhance psychoanalytic understanding. Just as important, everyday psychoanalytic conceptualizations, and the data from which they derive, can add considerably to the philosophies of mind and action. This is the case insofar as certain psychoanalytic concepts and data call out for philosophical explanation of contentful mental states that are clearly a-rational and irrational, whereas the usual domain for philosophy of mind and philosophy of action has been restricted to those mental states that are contentful and rational.[4]

Because in our work as psychoanalysts we have routine and fluid access to various primary process mediated mental states, states that are anything but rare, we can uniquely participate in the effort to understand cognitive (and conative) propositional attitudes[5] and mental states in general. In order to enlarge considerably the domain of philosophy of mind and philosophy of action by including these primary process states, we need to be clear about the differences among phantasies, beliefs-proper, and the more complex

---

[4] In fact there are many philosophers for whom the contentful mental states can only be rational. (See Cherniak 1981; Davidson 1970b, 1973, 1974, 1975, 1982; Dennett 1978, 1987; Fodor 1975, 1986; and Stich, 1983.) These philosophers are meaning holists who do allow for the occasional irrational contentful mental state, but only in the context of generalized normative rationality. I have taken issue with this view and I have presented a positive case for primary process (a-rational) mental states with referring representational content in Chapter 5, a revised version of Brakel (2002).

[5] Cognitive propositional attitude contents concern that which is the case—for example, I believe that X is coming toward me now; whereas conative propositional attitude contents concern that which is to be made the case—for example, I desire for X to come toward me now. More about cognitive and conative attitudes will follow below and in Chapter 8.

category of neurotic-belief. I shall begin with three examples of neurotic-beiefs. I hope to demonstrate two points with these examples. First, although neurotic-beliefs do not meet the criteria (to be elaborated at length below) for beliefs-proper at all, they are subjectively experienced no differently from beliefs-proper. Second, that the phenomenon of experiencing neurotic-beliefs as beliefs-proper is so prevalent, it can be demonstrated with almost any psycho-analytic patient in any hour. Thus what follows are accounts of the neurotic-beliefs of my first three patients on the day I wrote (the first draft of) this section.

Three patients with neurotic-beliefs on an ordinary psychoanalytic morning

Ms A

My first patient, Ms A, a 67-year-old administrator of a multi-specialty law firm, began the session lamenting her lack of authority. She was aware that her voice was barely audible, and she complained that her clothes were nonde-script and her overall appearance mousy. She felt terrible, as if she were some-one in hiding. We recognized these as familiar complaints. They arose from her acting upon her *neurotic-belief* that there was just one way to prevent a present day recurrence of the very damaging sexual behavior her father engaged in with her when she was between the ages of three and eleven years. Namely, Ms A always hid and made herself unappealing so that all men would keep their distance. "Evidence" confirming her neurotic-belief was brought to bear. She reported that her current behavior has in fact lead to no inappropriate sexual relationships; although unfortunately to no satisfying ones either. Then with respect to the past, Ms A evinced some psychic-reality-based "knowl-edge." Ms A "knew" that since neither of her younger sisters, both of whom were neglected and hence disheveled, nor her chronically ill mother *attracted* her father in the same way she did, it must have been that Ms A, a very pretty three-year-old much desiring her father's affection, was herself responsible for her father's acts.[6] So she "knew" she should have made herself hidden and unappealing then too. And Ms A neurotically believed, via a primary process conflation of past with present, that she had best remain that way now. Ms A experienced these neurotic-beliefs as beliefs-proper and she acted on

---

[6] Note that there is no indication in the transference or by report that Ms A. had been a seductive or sexually provocative child.

them—hiding from men and making herself unappealing—just as she would act if they were beliefs-proper.[7]

But they are not beliefs-proper, not even false ones, as there is no adjusting their content in accord with considerations of reality and truth. Ms A's neurotic-beliefs are more like complex primary process organized phantasies central to her neurotic problem; phantasies in which reality-based evidence seeking and attempts to regulate content toward truth and knowledge are replaced by a façade of psychic-reality-based "knowledge."

Dr B

My second patient, Dr B is a 55-year-old family practitioner. He was raised in a family in which he felt cared about and important, with a doting and admiring although sometimes inattentive father, and a "know-it-all" "do-it-my-way" mother. Although he realizes his parents were in no way actually rejecting, he has always felt he's been a disappointment to each of them. This is related to a *neurotic-belief* he holds on to: namely, that everyone who is important to him finds him unattractive, physically and emotionally.[8] Thus, Dr B took the better part of this session to recount an impressively long list of friends, colleagues, patients, and persons who were potential love interests, all of whom had, via phone, e-mail, regular mail, or directly, complimented him on his looks and/ or qualities of character. We were used to this; and he commented that he was still trying to test reality by amassing evidence to counter his standard view of himself. But as we both understood, this endeavor, no matter how many times repeated, would likely be useless. It was mere reality-tested evidence; and this had had no sway with Dr B's psychic-reality "knowledge." Dr B's cognitive attitude here is a neurotic-belief not a belief-proper and therefore no amount of evidence to the contrary will count toward falsifying and then dropping it.

---

[7] Ms A was not always conscious of the contents of her neurotic-belief; nor was she often aware of the "evidence" she gathered to "confirm" it. Usually neurotic-beliefs are not fully conscious. Part of the work of psychoanalysis is to infer from rigidly repetitive behaviors (such as Ms A's) the contents of a neurotic-belief and its components, including both the central unconscious phantasy and whatever psychic-reality-testing keeps it in place. The next step is to bring both aspects together for the patient to experience in conscious awareness. However, even when patients become aware of the whole operation, neurotic-beliefs remain extremely resistant to change.

[8] Unlike the case with most neurotic-beliefs (see footnote 7), Dr B has been quite conscious of the content of this one since the beginning of his treatment.

Mr C

Patient three, Mr C, a 26-year-old married architect, was intermittently intense or withdrawn in his relationship to his wife. We learned, owing to a very recent and acrimonious fight they had, that whenever she felt her need for space compromised (as she often did), he felt her to be rejecting him with much force. He could not tolerate being excluded by her and felt the need to make it right immediately, which was of course impossible. Mr C next had the following associations. Yesterday, after the session, he had been able to think about our work together for some 15 minutes after the session. He realized that, although remarkable, rarely had he had any thoughts whatever about his analysis between sessions; and in fact he stopped his participation about one minute before the scheduled ending time of each appointment. Today we were able to understand why he withdrew before I ended each session, and why he stayed withdrawn until we began the next one. This behavior owed to a *neurotic-belief* that my stopping each hour constituted a rejection; and that rather than live through the 24 hours or so until our next appointment, he made our relationship nonexistent.

I speculated too (although not yet with my patient), that the revival of our relationship every day was an important transference manifestation of one of his most central and longed-for phantasies—a phantasy contributing to another neurotic-belief, namely that his relationship with his long dead mother could likewise be revived so regularly and so easily. When I do discuss this with him, I will likely talk in terms of my patient's "acting as though he believes" that the dead-then-alive cycle in the analytic hours is something he can recreate with his mother, thereby bringing her back to life, if only temporarily. I will make the interpretation without expecting a change in my patient's thinking either on the basis of reality-based knowledge about the nature of death or, on what will be his new knowledge about the neurotic-belief he maintains. And yet, I will comment to Mr C in terms of his *"acting as though he believes"* because he will not experience the contents of such a neurotic-belief in any way different from how he would experience the contents of a belief-proper.

The neurotic-beliefs of Ms A, Dr B, and Mr C are different both from religious and social beliefs, which need admit of no evidential modifications, and from beliefs-proper which must be reality-tested and rendered true or false. Note that for all three patients the contents of the neurotic-beliefs discussed here are closely related to each patient's core phantasies. But this should not be taken to mean that phantasies are the same as neurotic-beliefs. Phantasies (as I will discuss at greater length later) are often at least partly unconscious, primary process based, and prior to considerations of reality-testing and truth vs. falsity. Neurotic-beliefs are composed of one or more phantasies, *plus* psychic-reality-based "knowledge" which provides confirming "evidence" for the phantasies' content, affording the neurotic-belief holder what seems to him/her like a secondary process/rational experience. Neurotic-beliefs can in this way be considered "phantasies-plus."

The following analogy might clarify this further. A *phantasy* bears the same relationship to a *neurotic-belief* that a *latent dream wish distorted by the primary process dream work* does to a *manifest dream*. Both neurotic-beliefs and manifest dreams need their façades of secondary process rationality.[9]

As for phantasies themselves—including the sort of structured, complex, partly unconscious, multileveled and multi-determined type of phantasy described in these three patients—they too are quite different from beliefs-proper. Just how they are different and why they are different is of central importance and will be addressed forthwith.[10]

Definitions of belief-proper and phantasy

A belief-proper, in philosophical terms, is that type of cognitive propositional attitude that aims at the truth. (See Velleman 1998, 2000, p.16.) Thus, Ms A cannot have the belief-proper "it is time for my Monday session to end" unless she has reason to think that the particular set of conditions obtains by which this proposition would be true—namely that this is a Monday and that this session started at 9:45 a.m. and it is now 10:30 a.m. The content of a belief is regulated with respect to truth considerations. What this amounts to is that the contents of beliefs-proper are specified in real time and place, and these contents are always (and ever) subjected to reality-testing with respect to their truth conditions as matched with what obtains in the real world. Thus she can maintain her belief-proper that it is time for the session to end now, November 21, 2005 at 10:30 a.m. in Ann Arbor, even when she remembers that it is 8:30 a.m. in Colorado, where she grew up. On the other hand, if Ms A has the belief-proper that the session will momentarily end, but consults her watch (which is in good working order) to find that it is 10:10 a.m., she will no longer hold the

---

[9] See Chapter 4.

[10] I will not, however, take up the very interesting and complicated story of how phantasies, particularly unconscious phantasies embodying various important unconscious conflicts, become structured and organized as central to the formation and maintenance of individual neuroses. This area, to provide but a very incomplete list, has been amply and ably discussed in the literature from the classic works of Freud (see especially (1905a [1901]), 1906 [1905], 1909, 1916, and 1919), to the modern extension of this view by Arlow (1985, 1991a, 1991b, and 1996), and with respect to developmental considerations by Novick and Novick (1996).

belief-proper that the session is about to end. Moreover, because the belief-proper with the content "the session will be ending now" would under these conditions entail a contradiction, not only will she no longer hold this belief, she *can* no longer hold it—at least not as a belief-proper. Obviously she can still desire, wish, or phantasize that the session were ending; and any of these may have had a causal role in the initial, but now known to be false, belief. But what Ms A cannot do is hold the belief-proper that the session will end now, while knowing that it will not. Beliefs-proper are propositional attitudes that are examples of secondary process mentation; they are each grounded in a particular time and place, they are all reality-tested, and regulated with respect to these truth considerations, and they do not admit of contradictions.[11] All of this requires some cognitive sophistication and maturity.

Let us now apply these criteria for belief-proper to the neurotic-beliefs of my three patients. Take first that beliefs-proper must be specified in terms of time and place. Ms A has a neurotic-belief that the way to stop men (who all are equivalent to her father) from engaging in inappropriate sexual relations with her is to make herself into a mousy hidden person. This is a propositional attitude in which the present is confused with the past. While being a less-appealing little girl, she might (questionably) have deterred her father's patho-logical sexual interests, being a mousy woman will do nothing to stop what happened in the past. Yet Ms A's neurotic-belief operates in a tenseless and unexamined present; it functions more like a phantasy (as we will see just below).

Now what about the reality-testing criterion for beliefs-proper? Dr B's case demonstrates that even though he accepts evidence that he is an attractive person, contrary to his neurotic-belief that he is not, his neurotic-belief remains every bit as fixed. His neurotic-belief both admits of contradiction and is not subject to reality-testing.

Similarly, Mr C's neurotic-belief that I reject him and abandon him in stopping each session is impervious to evidence to the contrary, and thereby tolerates contradiction. Further, with this neurotic-belief he conflates the present with the past, enacting in the "revival" of our relationship every day, a desired

---

[11] Yet it is obvious that people frequently have contradictory beliefs. In fact as long as the believer is unaware of the inconsistency, contradictory beliefs are maintained with no particular problem. However, whenever a rational person holding a belief-proper is made aware of a contradictory belief-proper, he/she will not tolerate the inconsistency. One belief or the other is dropped or modified, or perhaps both are modified, such that no conscious contradiction is allowed to stand.

revival of a relationship with a loved one long deceased. It is obvious that none of these neurotic-beliefs meet any of the criteria for beliefs-proper.

Phantasies are also quite different from beliefs-proper. From a philosophical perspective the difference is appreciated in that phantasies are characterized as those cognitive propositional attitudes[12] in which there are no attempts to match the truth conditions of the proposition to what obtains in the world. (See Chapter 5, and Brakel 2002.) Thus, if Ms A has longed for a break from the work of her analysis, she might phantasize that "It is at least 10:30 a.m. now in Ann Arbor and this session will very soon end for today"[13] without any consideration of the actual time. Moreover, even if she is made aware that the time in Ann Arbor is now only 10:10 a.m., her phantasy that it is at least 10:30 a.m. can remain her phantasy because phantasies, unlike beliefs-proper, can admit contradictions with reality. Further, phantasies are different from beliefs-proper with respect to time and place specifications too. Thus, Ms A can phantasize that her drive away from my office which will occur at 10:35 a.m. is happening right now; or that since it would be the case that if she were in Paris it would be around 3:10 p.m., and 3:10 p.m. is many hours after her session, she can phantasize that many hours have passed since her session. Ms A could even phantasize that she is in London; and that Ann Arbor is on London time as a new division of London. Finally, not only can phantasies admit of truth conditions that do not match up with what obtains in the world, they can be inconsistent with one another (as above), and each phantasy can even have contents that are internally contradictory. Thus Ms A can phantasize both that she is working in her psychoanalytic session now, and that co-temporaneously she is taking a break from psychoanalysis, enjoying the London afternoon. If Ms A should happen to become aware of the contradiction and want to "correct" it, she can create a phantasy with a condensation: she can phantasize,

---

[12] The notion of phantasies as contentful cognitive attitudes is controversial. The argument for phantasies having representational content is developed at length in Chapter 5 (and Brakel, 2002). With respect to phantasies as *cognitive* attitudes, although (as will be addressed below) they contain an embedded fulfilled wish, where the wish is a conative attitude, from the view of the phantasizer, contents of phantasies concern the *state of affairs as they are*, as is the case with all cognitive attitudes. (The contents of conative attitudes are concerned instead with *making states of affairs some certain way*.)

[13] From this very simple example a very important difference between the cognitive attitude, phantasy, and the conative attitude, wish can be seen. A phantasy, even in its most basic form, always has mental content such that a wish (or set of wishes) is represented as fulfilled, for example, the content represents *something that is the case*. Wishes, as a conative attitude type, represent *something that is to be brought about*. Thus wishes can exist in unfulfilled, not-yet-fulfilled, and even unfulfillable forms.

for example, us together in London, analyzing but also having a break from analysis. Clearly, in psychoanalytic terms, phantasies, even the conscious phantasies of adults, conform much more to primary process type mentation. Phantasies are not reality-tested; they do not rely on time and place specifications, instead taking place in the "tenseless and unexamined present"; and they admit of contradictions (or primary process condensation "corrections" for contradictions) quite readily.

Preliminary developmental considerations

If it is correct to categorize beliefs-proper as examples of secondary process mentation, then the capacity to hold beliefs-proper necessitates that any holder of such has achieved a great deal of cognitive development. After all, the capacity for secondary process mental operations requires much of thinkers. Mental contents need to be specified in terms of a particular and correct time and place. Contradictions must be appreciated, then not tolerated. Finally, the state of affairs obtaining in the world must be matched with the set of truth conditions that can make specific propositions true. In psychoanalytic terms these capacities constitute the general ability to test reality.

Because phantasies are propositional attitudes of a primary process nature, they do not require as much cognitive sophistication. In fact young children can have contentful[14] phantasies well before any consideration of truth and falsity, any constraining time variables, any attempt to test reality, and any notion of contradiction. But of course phantasies are phantasized not just by the very young not yet capable of beliefs-proper. Phantasies are also phantasized by cognitively mature adults. When an adult has a phantasy, he/she has consciously or unconsciously suspended the need to exclude contradictions and to specify time and place—he/she is no longer testing reality. Thus, a phantasy is marked either by the developmental incapacity for, or the suspension of, these interrelated abilities.

That this is unique to phantasizing among the cognitive propositional attitude types becomes apparent when we look not only at phantasy vs. belief-proper, but at several other cognitive attitude types including hypothesizing, supposing, imagining, and pretending. Each of these others, even pretending, depends on the capacity for assessing truth conditions of the proposition in question, and the related capacity for ascertaining whether these have been met, so that the proposition can be judged as true or false. In psychoanalytic

---

[14] Again, by contentful I mean mental content that is *about* something; namely that the mental content represents and refers to something.

terms, even pretending is preceded by the exercise of secondary process reality-testing (including time and place orientation) with regard to matching what is pretended with conditions obtaining in the world. Thus, Mr C, who with his young son, pretends to be a dinosaur in the dinosaur age, cannot really pretend this without the prior background understanding that he is a human father in the post-dinosaur era.[15]

Imagining, is a thought-dominated type of pretending, of which there are two forms. The first is a straightforward mental pretending in which for example, I cannot imagine spreading my wings and taking flight unless I understand that I am a flightless bipedal creature with two arms, two legs, and no wings. In this type of imagining, just as is the case with pretending, what I suspend is not the capacity for reality-testing and truth vs. falsity assessment, but the conclusions from these operations after I have performed them. In the other type of imagining, although there is no suspension of reality-testing capacities, tests of reality have not yet been performed and one may even choose not to perform them. Thus, I can imagine that X, my former supervisor, is at the gym today, without checking, and without wanting to check. Pretending and both types of imagining are very different from phantasizing because in phantasizing the very *capacities* for truth/falsity assessment, time/space assignment, and reality-testing are either not yet in place or have been suspended. Further, in phantasizing the suspension can take place either under one's conscious direction or unconsciously, whereas with pretending and both types of imagining reality-testing operations (or products thereof) are actively and consciously put to the side.

---

[15] Wimmer and Perner (1983) did a classic experiment showing that the ability to pretend comes after the ability to form beliefs-proper. Children were shown a puppet play in which a puppet named Maxi first puts some candies in a box and then goes out to play. While he is out playing the mother puppet moves the candies to the cupboard. Children are asked where Maxi will look for the candies on his return. Five-year-olds have no trouble indicating that Maxi will look for the candies in the box where he left them. But three- and four-year-olds more often indicate that Maxi will look for the candies in the cupboard. These children have a correct belief-proper that the candies are in the cupboard, where the mother puppet has put them, but they cannot pretend to be in Maxi's position; they cannot pretend to be in the position of one who does not have this belief-proper.

As interesting as these findings are, this experiment should not be taken to indicate that the ability to pretend is an all-or-none ability. Rather, what is suggested is that while all three groups of children showed the capacity for true beliefs-proper, the five-year-olds demonstrated the capacity for sophisticated pretending more than did the three- and four-year-olds.

The distinction between phantasizing and the second type of imagining can be tricky. How can we distinguish between *choosing to suspend one's capacity for reality-testing* in having a phantasy that X is at the gym vs. *choosing not to reality-test* the imagination that X is at the gym? I contend that there is an important difference. In the example of imagining something, the imaginer is always aware not only of what is imagined but also of "imagining," of having a particular type of propositional attitude, an imagination. In phantasizing something, however, once one has suspended (consciously or unconsciously) reality-testing capacity, one is aware only of the content of the phantasy, not of the particular propositional attitude "phantasizing." This is the reason that people often get lost in their phantasies (or daydreams); but seldom in their imaginings. To further fill out this distinction, take entities that cannot exist— impossible geometrical figures, the current King of France, a golden mountain, and so on. These impossible entities can be imagined or phantasized. When I imagine these entities, I am aware that I am imagining, and because I am aware that I am imagining (and not having beliefs-proper) I am also aware that these entities are impossible. When I phantasize about these same impossible entities, since genuine phantasizing requires either the suspension or insufficient development of reality-testing capacities, I am aware only of these entities—entities that happen to be impossible—while I have no awareness of the reality status of these entities, nor that the propositional attitude I am engaging in is "phantasizing." (See the following section, and the section on dream-beliefs for fuller explanations.)

Supposing and hypothesizing are even more sophisticated with respect to truth and reality-testing. With supposing, the truth conditions of the proposition are stipulated as being met by what obtains in the world—that is, the supposition is taken-as-true—without emphasis on investigating whether or not it is true. Suppositions are supposed-true for some purpose, for example, in order to further an exploration, make an argument, continue a discussion, and so on. The capacity to test reality is quite intact. However, reality-testing is put off, with the truth of the proposition presumed temporarily in order to further some more pressing goal. With hypothesizing that some proposition is true, there is not only the presupposition that hypothesizers possess intact capabilities for assessing truth and falsity and can reality-test, but also that they have serious interests in the truth status of the propositions in question. Hypothesizers are concerned with getting things right with respect to the propositions and their relations to the state of affairs of the world. They have perhaps performed some reality-testing operations already. And they will likely be interested in the outcome of other, more definitive tests. Note that agents who are making suppositions and those who are hypothesizing are quite aware that these are the cognitive attitudes they are employing.

A two-stage development of two reality-testing skills

By examining these different cognitive propositional attitudes, we can see that a two-stage cognitive development with respect to truth assessment and reality-testing takes place. The capacity for phantasizing marks the first stage in the development of propositional attitudes with truly representational, referring mental content (see Brakel 2002, chapter 5). The earliest in this series of propositional attitudes, phantasizing, does not require the capacity to test reality, nor to provide time/place specifications, nor to discern truth from non-truth. Phantasies take place before such reality constraints can be appreciated and before the difference between truth and non-truth can be considered.

Not so with pretending and imagining, two types of cognitive attitudes with which phantasies are often confused. These are cognitive propositional attitudes belonging to the second stage of development. Here, contrasts between the situations pretended and those in the world are registered, and pretenders and imaginers must be able to assess the match between truth conditions of the particular propositions pretended and the particular affairs obtaining in the world. This is true reality-testing, a skill (more properly a collection of skills) necessary for genuine pretending or imagining.[16] The operations of reality-testing are suspended, or the outcome of the reality tests are overruled, only insofar as, for the person pretending/imagining, aims more important than reality-testing and truth assessment continue to predominate. (Such aims can include, for instance, affect discharge, practice of skills, and just plain fun.)

There is another reality-testing skill differentiating those at the second stage of reality-testing development from those at the first. Unlike phantasizers, imaginers and pretenders, and certainly supposers[17] and hypothesizers are aware that they are imagining, pretending, supposing, or hypothesizing. Thus on any specific occasion, to pretend, imagine, suppose, or hypothesize some content requires not just a grasping of that content, but correct cognitive attitude typing with respect to the vehicle of that content. Further, those who are actively pretending, imagining, supposing, and hypothesizing must be

---

[16] Analogously, Novick and Novick (2000) hold that playing is not really possible without an understanding that the play differs from real life, in other words, that the play is play (p. 203).

[17] Supposing can be considered an intellectual type of imagining and pretending. As with pretending and the first type of imagining, something, p, can be supposed-as-true, even when the supposer knows p to be not true. As with the second type of imagining, something, p, can be supposed-as-true even choosing not to investigate p's relation to truth or falsity.

aware that the particular cognitive attitude type involved is different from belief-proper.

What developmental level of reality-testing is shown by my three patients in holding their neurotic-beliefs? It is clear that all three patients mistype their neurotic-beliefs as beliefs-proper, experiencing them as such. This is despite the fact that truth assessment, time/place specification, and reality-testing necessary for beliefs-proper do not take place. Instead, their neurotic-beliefs are fueled by the positive "evidence" supplied by psychic-reality, with the very activity of "evidence" seeking, as well as the "confirmation" accrued, contributing to each of these patients' subjective experience of their neurotic-beliefs as beliefs-proper. And yet, despite these secondary process operations, the neurotic-beliefs reflect developmental reality-testing functioning at the same early developmental level as phantasies.

Connections with conative propositional attitudes: Wishes and desires

So far we have been looking at the cognitive capacities sufficient for phantasies as compared with the more advanced cognitive capacities necessary for beliefs-proper. For the latter several capabilities characteristic of secondary process mentation are needed: (1) reality-testing consisting in matching propositional truth conditions with what obtains in the world, (2) the ascription of truth vs. non-truth, and (3) the ability to classify the type of cognitive propositional attitude one is employing. All three of these higher level, secondary process capacities are absent in phantasizing, but present (at least to some extent) in pretending and imagining, and fully operative in supposing, hypothesizing, and believing-proper.

But how do the conative propositional attitudes of wishing and desiring fit here? Although it might be obvious that wishes belong with phantasies and beliefs belong with desires, the criteria we used to distinguish between the two stages of development in the cognitive propositional attitudes will not be of much use here. Wishes can be contradictory, they are impervious to constraints of reality-testing, and truth conditions for these propositions do not even make sense. One cannot say, for instance, that the content of a wish is true or not true. But all of this is no less the case for desires.[18] I can desire to be an eager, fresh eight-year-old again, fully knowing it will never happen.

---

[18] In Chapter 8, I will make a case for "readiness-to-act" as the constitutive function of desire; this being the basis for distinguishing desire from wish as a distinct conative attitude type.

Further, I can desire to be eight years old again and, at the same time desire to be as wise and knowledgeable and old as the most senior analyst or philosopher.

However, before we abandon these familiar criteria, let us note that the very same secondary process capacities—the many aspects of reality-testing, for example—are often used by desire-ers, but not about the desire itself. Rather, desire-ers use reality-testing to assess cognitive attitudes relevant to fulfilling their desires. Thus a person with a desire, unlike a person with a wish (1) will often evaluate whether on matters pertaining to the desire's fulfillment, there is a match between what obtains in the world and his/her beliefs-proper, and (2) will regulate the latter to conform to reality. These two steps take place for the purpose of developing some plan of action to fulfill the desire. Simply put, people often use reality-tested, secondary process beliefs-proper to act in such a way as to maximize chances to satisfy their desires.[19] For an everyday example, suppose Dr B gets a message from his secretary that an old friend from out of town is here in Ann Arbor for one day only and wants to meet him at 2 p.m. Suppose further that on this day Dr B has a full load of patients scheduled, and his analytic appointment is at 2 p.m. He has, given the realities of time and space, what amount to contradictory desires: to meet his friend at 2 p.m., and to see his analyst at 2 p.m. But by having various consistent beliefs-proper he can choose a course of action to attempt to maximize the fulfillment of both of these desires. Suppose he has a belief-proper that despite his secretary's message about his friend's specific availability, his friend is usually rather flexible about time. Or suppose he remembers that his analyst occasionally has been able to reschedule on short notice, so that he has the belief-proper that she might be able to now. Dr B can put these beliefs-proper to the test and try to rearrange one of the 2 p.m. meetings. On the other hand, suppose Dr B held a different belief-proper about his friend, namely, that although possessing many good qualities, he is given to playing stupid jokes on people. Or suppose Dr B noted that his own secretary had been making a lot of mistakes lately in taking phone messages. In neither of these last two instances would he yet have a sufficient set of beliefs-proper to warrant changing his original schedule, despite really desiring to see his friend.

The situation with wishes is much different. Wishes seek fulfillment too, but a different cognitive attitude, phantasizing, is most closely associated with

---

[19] Someone with a desire uses beliefs-proper in order to act so as to maximize opportunities for desire satisfaction. As will be taken up in Chapter 8, this is just one way that desire can be linked to action, manifesting its "readiness-to-act." Wishes are not marked by readiness-to-act; furthermore wishes employ phantasizing as the cognitive attitude vehicle for their fulfillment, not beliefs-proper. This last will be addressed below.

their satisfaction. Clearly, phantasies will not admit of reality-testing. And because phantasies play a very different role in satisfying wishes from that played by beliefs-proper with respect to desires, tests of reality would be anything but useful anyway. To illustrate the operation of wish and phantasy, take for example my patient Mr C and the wish he sometimes has to be both male and female. In his phantasy of this state, he *is* two; one who is male and one who is female. And he has two other separate phantasies, one where he is male, and another where he (she) is female. There is no problem that the first phantasy is internally inconsistent and that the two subsequent ones are inconsistent with one another. There is no problem that both of these wishes are impossible given the real world of earth physics and normal human biology. It is in using these phantasies as a vehicle that his wishes are experienced (phantasized) as fulfilled.

Beliefs-proper, unlike phantasies, must be independent of desires and wishes

In their relationship to the conative attitudes, there is an important difference between beliefs-proper and phantasies—a difference in which the two-stage development concerning primary process vs. secondary process capacities is central. Beliefs-proper must be held (or dropped) irrespective of desires (and wishes), according instead to the truth conditions obtaining in the world. No matter how much she desires to be in London, when a nonpsychotic person like Ms A sees a university building from my office window she must hold the belief-proper that she is seeing a part of the University of Michigan in Ann Arbor, not the London School of Economics in London. And, no matter how appealing Mr C would find it to be both male and female, no matter how he wishes for such an omnipotent state, the real-world evidence that he is a man necessitates that he cannot hold the content "I am male and female" as a belief-proper. He can wish that this were so; he can phantasize that it is so; but he cannot hold a belief-proper that he is male and female, as there is much reality-tested real-world evidence to the contrary.[20]

On the other hand, there is no need whatever for phantasies to be independent from wishes (and desires). In fact it is reasonable to wonder if phantasies can even exist without some embedded conative attitude. Could Mr C have a

---

[20] He has at times held the neurotic-belief that he is part male and part female, with reality-testing supplanted by the psychic-reality "evidence" that his hips and skin are really feminine in character.

phantasy of being male and female without this phantasy representing some sort of wish or set of wishes?

To be capable of having the type of cognitive propositional states (i.e. beliefs-proper) that are entirely separate from conative propositional states (i.e. wishes and desires), secondary process mediated reality-testing must have developed sufficient stability that it will be maintained even under the pressures of wishes and desires to override it. An interesting example of reality-testing which is not so sturdy comes from an experiment with chimps reported in the journal *Science*. (The work was done by Sarah Boysen at Ohio State University as reported by Fishman 1993.)

Chimps were trained until each had the ability to recognize the plastic Arabic numerals, "1" through "10," and to associate these numerals with the number of items indicated. This ability, which included the understanding of more vs. fewer items, was demonstrated as follows. There was an initial training on numerals and their associated number amounts. One chimp then had several runs in which she was given a choice of two plastic numerals, for example, a "4" and an "8"—with one of the numerals to represent the number of gum-drops she would get, and the other to represent the number of food bits for her partner, another chimp. One numeral was always higher than the other. The selecting chimp picked the higher plastic numeral first (e.g. "8"), got rewarded with eight gumdrops, and then watched her partner chimp get the four gum-drops represented by the remaining plastic "4." Next, a new and more compli-cated condition was introduced for the chimp pairs. Reporting on a typical pair, Sarah the selecting chimp and Sheba her partner, the experimenters now gave Sheba, the partner chimp, the number of gumdrops matching the numeral Sarah, the selecting chimp, chose first. Thus when Sarah chose the plastic "7," Sheba got seven gumdrops and Sarah herself was left with the plastic "3" and three gumdrops. After a number of such trials Sarah had no trouble picking the lower valued plastic numeral first, thereby reserving for herself the higher numeral and the larger number of gumdrops represented. From the experiment-ers' view (really from any view) the learning experiment was a great success.

But a control condition is of interest for our purposes. When, instead of the plastic numerals, the experimenters used two piles with differing numbers of gumdrops—for example, four gumdrops vs. eight gumdrops—Sarah, the chimp flawlessly making the plastic numeral selections so as to increase her own gumdrop reward, could not learn to forestall choosing the pile with more gumdrops first. Presumably an easier task in that no association of numeral with number is required, Sarah could not help but choose the pile with the greater number of gumdrops first, even after seeing that again and again Sheba rather than Sarah got the big gumdrop pay off. It seems Sarah could not stop the desire for more food from interfering with aspects of her reality-testing capacities. She could not separate her secondary process mediated belief-proper that she would get the bigger pile if and only if she first pointed to the smaller pile, from her primary process desire for as much of the obviously available food *now*! The independence of her cognitive states from her conative states was overridden. It failed under the pressure of the chimp's increased desire for the gumdrops. Her desire was intensified by the increased visibility of the gumdrops, which seemed to signal an immediate availability that proved irresistible.

Back in the human world, my patients' neurotic-beliefs are also not independent of wishes and desires. Ms A's neurotic-belief that her hidden, nondescript appearance will ward off future inappropriate sexual advances cannot be separated from her longstanding primary process wishful desire that such a presentation to the world would have had a protective effect in the past. Nor can this same neurotic-belief be isolated from her current, and equally primary process-mediated (almost magical) wishful desire that she was never in fact abused. Similarly, Mr C's neurotic-belief that I stop the sessions intending to reject him cannot exist: (1) without his concurrent desire (and preemptive action) to be the one who stops our relationship, and (2) without the older wishes (upon which the present day desire and behavior are predicated) to never have felt and never feel again the pain of being abandoned by his mother.

The realm of action: Beliefs-proper, phantasies, neurotic-beliefs, and dream-beliefs

Beliefs-proper and action

To this point, three important differences between phantasies and beliefs-proper have been discussed. First, the conditions under which the contents of beliefs-proper are true or false must be assessed with respect to conditions in the world. This reality-testing skill is not required for phantasies. Second, having a belief-proper necessitates being capable of properly distinguishing beliefs-proper from other cognitive attitudes. No such capability for correctly typing cognitive attitudes is required for phantasies. Third, beliefs-proper must be assessed with independence from attendant desires and wishes—they must be retained or dropped based solely on matches between their content and the state of affairs obtaining in the world, with wishes and desires having no influence. This is not required for phantasies; on the contrary most (all) phantasies consist of embedded wishes experienced as fulfilled.

In this subsection I will illustrate with an example that beliefs-proper, *because* they require (1) reality-testing, (2) propositional attitude recognition, and (3) the separation of cognitive from conative attitudes, serve as a better ground for actions than do phantasies. Further, this superiority is so pronounced, that a privileged relationship between beliefs-proper and intentional actions is the default mode of operation for most of human behavior most of the time.

Here is the example directly contrasting beliefs-proper with phantasies as the grounds for action. Suppose I want to see a friend whom I last saw in New York City in 1968. We were fond of each other in those days, and he always welcomed my dropping in to visit day or night throughout our years of acquaintance. Grounding intentional actions on beliefs-proper, I would have to contact him to ascertain a number of things. Is my friend still alive and well? Would he be interested in my visiting after almost forty years? When would be a good time? Does he still live in New York, or somewhere else? If he is still in New York, does he live at the same address? If not New York, or if at a different address, where does he live? If he is alive, wants to see me, tells me his address, and suggests some time that would be good for a visit, I would, on the basis of these several beliefs-proper have sufficient grounds to plan a trip to visit him. Suppose, on the other hand, I have the very same desire to see him, but instead base my actions upon a set of phantasies, each with content to the effect that everything with my friend is unchanged. Without recognizing that I am phantasizing, I assume not only that he is alive and well, but that he is still at the same place, and that he would still enjoy a surprise visit from me. Suppose further that on the strength of these phantasies, without ever contacting him I book a flight to New York, take a bus to his old neighborhood, and then walk to his 1968 address. Which version of my trip is likely to end up well?

Clearly, actions based upon beliefs-proper seem better grounded than those predicated upon phantasies. This is a fact largely uncontested, certainly by patients in psychoanalysis, usually very competent and sane people. But what about actions predicated on neurotic-beliefs? What is the relationship of neurotic-belief to intentional action? Let us return to my three patients to investigate.

Neurotic-beliefs and action

Ms A's neurotic-belief that she must stay mousy leads her *to act* in countless numbers of ways every day. She walks with her head down, unsmiling and seldom making eye contact; she dresses so as to blend in; she stands stiffly upright to such an extent as to look uncomfortable; she speaks in a controlled, sometimes too loud, sometimes too soft, but always stilted fashion. Moreover, other than to conduct the essentials of her life, she does not get out much; she has few hobbies or interests, and certainly she has no fun. Consequent to these actions her life is without the pleasures of male friends, companions, and lovers.

Dr B's neurotic-belief that he is not attractive as a person, physically and emotionally, is painful. In fact so painful that he is driven *to act* by spending much of his waking time collecting people who think well of him in the hope of eventually disconfirming his entrenched neurotic-belief. He spends hours composing return e-mails, contemplating what people are thinking of him, and even asking the few friends he feels sure of what they think others are thinking about Dr B. At night he writes in his journal his worries about the various interactions he has had, both personally and professionally that day. Did he say the right thing? Was he firm enough? Did his advice make sense? Will person X still like him? He agonizes over his clothes, his hair, and whether or not he has aged badly, continually buying new clothes, getting his hair cut in different styles, and trying various anti-aging techniques. These neurotic-belief driven actions and behaviors, meanwhile, are obviously to the detriment of other actions and behaviors, which could potentially lead to the satisfying relationships for which Dr B longs.

Mr C's neurotic-belief that I reject him every day in ending the sessions also leads him *to act*. Namely, Mr C acts with the anticipatory counterattacks of terminating our relationship and ceasing all thoughts about his analysis from one minute before the end of every session until our work and relationship are revived the next day. These actions unchecked might have jeopardized the very analysis, and certainly do diminish its effectiveness. Likewise, his similar neurotic-belief that his wife is rejecting him if she seeks some space, leads Mr C to interact with her in several different ways—clinging and dependent, angrily provoking her rejection, or withdrawing first—each harmful to their marriage.

Why do these patients *act* on the basis of these neurotic-beliefs? The answer is that the neurotic-beliefs are experienced and treated as though they were beliefs-proper, and as such occupy the same privileged functional role with respect to action. Remember that in each case the neurotic-belief lead to actions only after psychic-reality-based "evidence" for its contents had been accrued. Thus, while contents of these neurotic-beliefs are actually the contents of primary process-mediated phantasies, they are (mis)taken for secondary process beliefs-proper. This is due in large part to the operation of psychic-reality-based searches for "evidence" and the resultant "confirmations." But this raises another vexing question. Granted that the search for evidence is an important secondary process operation—indeed the very notions of evidence and confirmation are secondary process concepts—why do primary process-mediated phantasies not just remain as primary process phenomena? Why does all of this secondary processing go on at all?

One answer comes directly from clinical theory: the secondary process façade stabilizes the underlying neurotic phantasy and increases its resistance to change. But in addition to this defensive process, there is a trait that can be regularly observed about human beings universally: once we are thinkers capable of secondary process thought, this more mature mode is used almost automatically almost all of the time to reinterpret and justify almost everything at every level. Secondary process predominates, especially in the alert–awake state of adults.[21] As was taken up in Chapter 4, this is partly why primary process is so hard to know. But as to why we secondary process thinkers do this (and here I must be more speculative), it seems that we like to think of ourselves as rational.[22] We like to think that we know what we are thinking, and we like to think that we know what we are doing.[23] And yet since the search for "evidence" for neurotic-beliefs is done based on psychic-reality, any chance for regulating the neurotic-beliefs according to truth/reality considerations has been corrupted. So we have people with phantasies, thinking that they have reality-tested them as they would beliefs-proper, resulting in neurotic-beliefs, not only resistant to change, but also with another serious consequence. The mistyping of neurotic-beliefs as beliefs-proper allows neurotic-beliefs to lead to intentional actions just the way beliefs-proper lead to intentional actions, often with very deleterious outcomes.

Reviewing reality-testing requirements for beliefs-proper

Beliefs-proper require reality-testing development that is at the second stage. This means that beliefs-proper must meet the four criteria for the second stage of reality-testing to qualify as actual beliefs-proper: (1) there must be an evaluative matching of the truth conditions of the content of beliefs-proper with the relevant conditions obtaining in the world, (2) there must be an ability to

---

[21] Further evidence for robust (perhaps overly robust) secondary processing will be given at the end of this chapter.

[22] Meaning holists would agree that we think of ourselves as largely rational. And for a subset of these philosophers, the attributionists, the condition of being largely rational is then charitably attributed to others as well.

[23] Velleman (1989, p.169) comes to the same conclusion about our liking to think we know what we are doing. He takes this up, however, more in terms of this desire shaping our actions rather than reinterpreting them: "an intellectual passion—our desire to know what we're doing—first restrains us from intending some actions we think we wouldn't understand and then encourages us to intend an action we that we think we would."

properly type cognitive attitudes such that the mental contents of beliefs-proper are regarded as the content of beliefs-proper, (3) beliefs-proper must be held (or dropped) independent from simultaneous desires and wishes, and (4) beliefs-proper, because of meeting the three criteria listed just above, bear a particular and privileged relationship to actions.

To appreciate more fully these four factors, it will prove useful to pursue propositional attitudes in a state different from alert awakeness. So, let us now examine various cognitive attitudes during dreaming.

Cognitive states and propositional attitudes in dreams, including dream-beliefs

The adult dream world seems to contain many of the cognitive states of the adult waking world, but within dreams. Adult dreamers, while dreaming, experience themselves as believing, imagining, pretending, supposing, perceiving, or remembering, and so on. But these dream-beliefs (and dream-perceivings, etc.) cannot really meet the criteria to be considered beliefs-proper (or veridical perceptions, etc.). Here is why. Although within the dream the dream-beliefs' contents presumably have been reality-tested against what obtains in the world, the world is a dream world and the reality-testing during dreams lacks the secondary process-mediated sophistication and consistency of awake world reality-testing. To illustrate, I present a dream I had while a medical student on an obstetrics rotation. It will be readily apparent why this dream belongs to a class of dreams Freud (1900, p.125) characterized as dreams of convenience: "I hear a loud clanging. I don't understand what it means but feel compelled to get up and go to the delivery room and assist, and so I go."

When I awakened I realized that in the dream I believed myself to have been present in the delivery room, when in actuality I was still in my "on-call" bed. In the awake state I also understood that the loud clanging, incomprehensible in my dream, had been my pager ringing, summoning me to the delivery room as the "on-call" medical student for the obstetrics service. Reality-testing even within the dream was off; and since in my dream I believed I had left for the delivery room, while in fact I slept soundly and dreamt, it is clear that my dream-belief did not help me match the truth conditions of the belief with what obtained in the world.

Like me, most dreamers are almost always incorrect when they, within their dreams, experience themselves to be having a belief-proper type of propositional attitude. Instead, dreamers are dreaming and believing-within-the-dream, that is, having dream-beliefs. But the great majority of dreamers in almost all of their dreams do not experience themselves as dreaming and therefore *cannot properly identify the type of propositional attitude* they employ.[24] Things do change as soon as the dreamer awakens. Once awake, most of the cognitive states and propositional attitudes of the dream can be properly ascribed. So the now awake dreamer, D, can say, "In my dream I remembered that X did A, B, C; but this was no memory, because X never did A, B, C, even though he wanted to." Or D can say, "All of those things I believed true of Z in the dream were not true at all. They came straight from my wishes about her." Also after awakening, dream-beliefs can be assessed as to whether or not their contents match that of (awake) beliefs-proper. For example, D, now awake, can say, "In my dream I believed that your hair was very long and green. Now, I still have the belief-proper that it is long, but of course it is not green."

Shevrin (1986, 1998) and I (Brakel 1989) debated about the role of consciousness in the ability to distinguish among the various types of cognitive states and propositional attitudes. Shevrin held that being *conscious-of* some mental content, whether it be the content of a dream, hallucination, or that of a conscious awake belief or memory, was sufficient to ascribe (and then fix or attach) the content to a particular cognitive state type (e.g. as a memory, perception, belief, wish, or an imagination, etc.). I, on the other hand, held that one's being *conscious-of* some content was necessary, but that the ascribing and attaching to a particular cognitive state type required *alert awake consciousness*. Dream-percepts and dream-beliefs make good counterexamples to Shevrin's claim. The mental content experienced as a visual percept in a dream might well never have been a percept. It can, for example, have had its origin as a memory or a daydream. As for a belief within a dream: (1) it may fail even the sketchy reality tests applicable within primary process dominated dreams, (2) it may reflect no waking belief-proper past or present of the dreamer, and (3) it cannot be properly identified within the dream as a dream-belief rather than a belief-proper. True, once awake from a dream or in a post-hallucinatory state, people can (most often) properly (re)-type the contents they had experienced as dream or hallucinatory contents in various cognitive state/propositional attitude forms. Yet even the grossest distinction—that between contents originating in a dream or hallucination vs. those originating in awake perceptions, memories, or beliefs—takes place only during alert consciousness. (And for sure, the finer discriminations that separate dream-percepts from awake percepts, and awake percepts both from awake images imagined and those remembered, will require alert awakeness.) Here then is a

---

[24] There are exceptions. Dreams in which dreamers have the thought: "I'm only dreaming" while not uncommon make up only a tiny fraction of remembered dreams.

simple example: "I had a dream in which X appeared in a full leg cast and I believed him to have broken his leg."

Only when I awakened did I realize X had not broken his leg; whereas within the dream, I erroneously experienced X's broken leg as a veridical percept and a belief-proper. Only in the subsequent alert wakeful condition did I properly type the dream-belief as having been a dream-belief. Further, only in alert wakefulness could I consider the dream-belief as revealing my phantasy (compete with fulfilled wish) of a broken legged X underlying and motivating the dream-belief.

This dream example provides another reason for revisiting the debate between Shevrin and me. That the correct cognitive state typing of the dream content can occur only after the dream, in the alert wakeful condition, demonstrates that proper discrimination among various cognitive and conative propositional attitudes requires another vital aspect of reality-testing. Mental content from attitudes that originate from inside must be recognized as such—for example, dream-percepts, hallucinatory-percepts, and wishes—and differentiated from propositional attitudes with content from the outside, for example, awake percepts and awake beliefs-proper that arise from these percepts. These distinctions are as impossible for dream-believers as they are for people having phantasies; the content of both dream-beliefs and phantasies consist in internal wishes somehow experienced as already fulfilled. Thus, during dreams dreamers regard the contents of their dream-beliefs as being the case—*from outside*, when in fact their contents are internal wishes in which something *from inside* is to be made the case.

It seems clear that dream-beliefs do not meet any of the criteria for beliefs-proper. Just to make sure, though, let us look at the four criteria for beliefs-proper to see if dream-beliefs can qualify on any of them. (1) It is clear from the foregoing that no dream-cognitive states can meet the reality-testing requirement of making the distinction between mental content from inside vs. that from outside, much less ascribing contents to the proper propositional attitude type. Even dream-beliefs, because they are dreamed as beliefs-proper, fail at both aspects of this reality-testing task. (2) Nor can dream-beliefs even match up the dream-beliefs' truth conditions with conditions obtaining in the world of the dream, much less those obtaining in the world. (3) In terms of the independence of cognitive states from conative states necessary for genuine beliefs-proper, dream-beliefs have no autonomy from underlying wishes and desires. As my dream of convenience shows, the dream-belief that I went to the delivery room is inextricably linked with my desire not to be awakened to work in the middle of the night. (4) Finally, do dream-beliefs have the same special relationship to actions that beliefs-proper do? Dream-beliefs do not.

During REM (Rapid Eye Movement) sleep volitional actions, routine and normal during waking states, cannot take place owing to a muscular paralysis normal for this sleep phase. The consequences of this can vary, but the vast majority of times this is in our best interest. So, while it is true that as I remained in bed asleep having the dream-belief that I was going to the delivery room, my reputation as a competent medical student was compromised; it is of far more significance that when Mr C dreamed that a thug was slugging him, with Mr C retaliating by taking out a knife and repeatedly stabbing the attacker, no one was physically harmed.[25]

Having examined the four criteria necessary for genuine belief-proper, a cognitive attitude requiring reality-testing development through the second stage, we can conclude that no dream-cognitive state or attitude, including dream-belief, can meet the criteria.

Confounds

Dream-beliefs and neurotic-beliefs are quite different from beliefs-proper. As we have seen, dreamers having dream-beliefs and persons with neurotic-beliefs are not able to test the reality of these cognitive attitudes, neither in terms of regulating their contents with respect to truth conditions in the world, nor with respect to proper cognitive attitude typing. And yet, very often neurotic-beliefs (and occasionally dream-beliefs) are acted upon as though they were genuine beliefs-proper, often with deleterious results. Earlier in this chapter the confounding of neurotic-belief for belief-proper was briefly addressed. But there are still aspects that warrant further consideration. For example, given that proper propositional attitude typing does not take place, why are the confusions in the direction of taking dream-beliefs and neurotic-beliefs to be beliefs-proper?

An answer to this question takes us back once more to the observation that awake, alert adult human thinkers consistently use rationally based secondary processes as the default mode of mental operation. We rely on basic principles of everyday logic such as noncontradiction, and various reality-testing skills. Hence in the service of putting content in a form that mature human thinkers find most workable—even if, as is the case with neurotic-beliefs, significant trouble arises from this transformation—much mental content from various

---

[25] There are individuals with REM Sleep Disorders in which they do act out their dreams with frightening results as if their dream beliefs were beliefs-proper. Patients, for instance, with dreams like Mr C's dream have been known to assault and physically harm their bed partners. (For a review article on this topic see Abad and Guilleminault, 2004.)

propositional attitude types is attributed in an incorrect, but reflex fashion to the propositional attitude belief-proper. Counting as evidence for this default operation is our human reaction to the cognitive world of toads, to which I now return yet again. (See Chapters 5 and 6.)

Toads, rapidly zip out their tongues whenever small black insects are within their visual fields. Toads are quite successful in capturing and then quickly swallowing these little black bugs, a not uninteresting fact. But more interesting still is that toads will repeatedly react in just the same way to small black lead pellets. They will zip out their tongues, capture, and swallow endless metal pellets or endless bugs, indiscriminately. What is going on for these toads? Is it, as many contend (including the philosophers, Dennett 1987 and Fodor 1986), that the toads (1) want bugs, (2) have beliefs-proper that black metal pellets are bugs, and therefore (3) go for every bug and metal pellet? If this were so, toads engaged in this behavior would be demonstrating the capacity to make correct inferences and to have genuine (albeit in this case false) beliefs-proper. Perhaps from this viewpoint the toad's cognitive problem would be diagnosed as an over-inclusive category for bug. The other alternative is that toads have a reflex-like reaction whenever a dark object of a certain size appears. If this is the correct explanation, when it comes to bugs and black metal pellets, successful toads probably have full bellies, but no beliefs-proper and no inference processes.[26]

But, despite the fact that the latter explanation requires far less speculative baggage, and is thereby a better bet, humans, once they have reached what has been referred to here as the second developmental stage, find imparting beliefs-proper and the capacity for beliefs-proper to others almost irresistible. Further, adult humans tend to attribute a full-blown capacity for genuine beliefs-proper not only to various creatures in the animal world,[27] but also to

---

[26] This sort of hard-wired reflex-like operation can certainly yield evolutionary success provided that over-inclusive eating of small black objects (1) does not prove toxic and (2) does not preclude the ingestion of real food. Indeed it should not be ruled out that toads have a genuine concept or category constituted by their reflex-like activity—a concept *we* might name "black things to capture and swallow." Note that as discussed in Chapter 6, from a toad's viewpoint such a category would not be over-inclusive. (See also Chapter 5, for a different view of the bug/metal pellet situation, in which toad representations of bug/metal pellets are shown to be genuine representations of bugs, but not metal pellets.)

[27] That toads are unlikely to have genuine beliefs-proper, in no way implies that toads are not capable cognizers. They can form percepts that are predictable and meaningful representations of the highly complex external world such that in conjunction with inputs from within, toads can perform actions, some instinctually driven, leading to biological

their own phantasy- and dream-states, as well as to very young children clearly not yet able to test reality.

More complex confounds

Neurotic-beliefs have an additional reason to be experienced and acted upon as though they were beliefs-proper. If, as I have proposed, neurotic-beliefs are core phantasies *plus* "evidence" and "confirmation" gained from psychic-reality-testing (as opposed to reality-testing), the natural tendency to ascribe contents to beliefs-proper in a default manner, will be strengthened by the performance of these distorted tests of reality. While it is a given that general reality-testing is not without its psychic-reality component and that therefore there is no reality that is not somewhat psychic-reality mediated, general reality-testing benefits from consensual objective world contributions modulating and even overruling many idiosyncratic psychic-reality verdicts.

The character of the "evidence" and "confirmation" gained to support neurotic-beliefs, on the other hand, makes clear that for this class of propositional attitudes, it is the conflict laden, primary process-organized psychic-reality-testing which predominates. Ms A, for instance, has "evidence" that since her own engaging behavior and appearance as a youngster caused (and will cause) men to abuse her, her mousy demeanor will prove protective. Dr B "knows" that he is not well liked. How does he know? Well it is because Persons X, Y, and Z, although responding to his communications did not do so warmly enough or strongly enough or quickly enough. And as for Mr C, his psychic-reality-testing "demonstrates" that everyday at the end of analytic sessions he is rejected by his analyst, most days rejected by his wife, and of course most painful of all, his mother rejected him by dying when he was quite young, impervious to his great need for her.

Note though that psychic-reality-testing performed on the contents of neurotic-beliefs *feels* no different from the reality-testing done for properly typed beliefs-proper; and that the "evidence" gathered from psychic-reality-testing is evaluated in the same manner as the evidence from regular reality-testing. Thus the holder of a particular neurotic-belief classifies it as a belief-proper,

---

success in terms of nutrition, survival, and reproduction. Toads can also learn, and as discussed in Chapter 5, it is certainly possible that they have concepts, categories, and the capacity for representational mentation. What I am questioning is the notion that toads can operate at the largely secondary process-mediated level necessary for genuine beliefs-proper. I speculate instead that their cognitive organization (including the sort of categories they form) is likely primary process mediated.

not only in accord with the default natural tendency to do so, but deliberately and with assurance! No wonder neuroses are so entrenched.

Consequences of the confounds

If beliefs-proper are attributed to toads when they really do not have the capacity for genuine beliefs, no harm is done. Of more importance is the tendency adults have to adultomorphize children. This arguably leads to unreasonable expectations and short parental patience, and certainly inhibits true empathic understanding. Relatedly, regarding aspects of our own mentation, we humans tend to assume more secondary process organization than is warranted in a number of ways. For example, we frequently assume that various awake cognitive states (including perceptions, memories, imaginations, beliefs, etc.) are independent of our conative states (wish, desire) when clearly they are not.[28] This assumption is closely related to one of the central theses of this chapter, namely that we often mis-(type) dream-cognitive states, waking complex phantasy states (which include underlying conflictual unconscious contents), and the "phantasy-plus" states of neurotic-beliefs, all as beliefs-proper. Looking generally at this sort of classification mistake, we can see it has far-reaching consequences. Because beliefs-proper, unique among the cognitive attitudes types, have privileged access to actions producing effects in the world, when mental contents in propositional attitudes other than beliefs-proper take over their functional role, actions and behaviors result which can be very harmful. What this amounts to is a very rudimentary account—derived from a philosophical analysis of various cognitive states and propositional attitudes— toward explaining why neuroses are so detrimental.

Before concluding, I want to make a practical point. The very classification mistake we have been examining here has resulted in raising unwarranted hopes about cognitive behavioral treatment. Indeed when it is the case that people are suffering from false beliefs-proper, cognitive behavioral therapy should (and often does) work. False beliefs-proper are genuine beliefs-proper, they just are wrong. But for many patients their problem is not one of erroneous

---

[28] For example, without even taking up the ubiquitous influence of unconscious and conflictual wishes and desires, it is clear that conscious desires have great influence not only on imaginations, memories, and beliefs, but also on basic perceptions. A very simple study by McClelland and Atkinson (1948) was done in which two groups of subjects— one group desiring food and very hungry and the other group not hungry—were asked to describe what they saw when they were presented what was actually just blobs or smudges on a screen. The hungrier group *saw* food items significantly more often than did the other group.

and false beliefs-proper. Rather, for these people, like my three patients, the problem is better characterized as four-layered: (1) there are unconscious conflicts involved in the content of the core, complex phantasy, (2) psychic-reality-testing (rather than reality-testing) yields "evidence" and distorted "confirmation" of the content of the phantasy, (3) there is a mistyping of the resultant neurotic-belief as a belief-proper, and (4) such neurotic-beliefs are experienced as beliefs-proper, and acted upon as such—as the functional role of these neurotic-beliefs aquires that of beliefs-proper. For problems of this sort no amount of cognitive behavioral therapy can work.

Perhaps an analog with the toad situation will help clarify why. If toads merely had the false belief-proper that metal pellets were bugs leading to an over-inclusive category, one would find that toads experienced with both bugs and metal pellets would after some training learn to modify the category and appreciate the difference. After all, on many external criteria to which toads are sensitive (taste, weight, texture), bugs are rather different from lead pellets. But toads will ingest countless numbers of both bugs and metal pellets, despite intensive and extensive "cognitive-behavioral" training attempts. Cognitive-behavioral training can change false and erroneous beliefs-proper. It cannot address a matter such as a hard-wired category born of a reflex-like proclivity to react to everything that is even potentially food. This is a matter at a different level. For each of my patients too, the problem is at a different level from that of false belief-proper. The complex, partly unconscious, multilevel, multi-determined, central phantasies *plus* the psychic-reality-testing derived "confir-mation" of their content—the neurotic-beliefs that Ms A, Dr B, and Mr C each experience as beliefs-proper—are not simply false beliefs-proper. These are neurotic-beliefs—not beliefs-proper at all. Treatment attempting to address these phantasy laden, primary process-mediated, neurotic-beliefs as though they were false beliefs-proper, will be a misguided treatment precisely *because* such treatment would be predicated on one of the very sources of the problem—the mistyping of cognitive propositional attitudes that are not beliefs-proper as beliefs-proper.

Conclusion

This chapter has interdisciplinary aspirations in two directions. In one direc-tion, using philosophical technical definitions along with the philosophical method of making concise and consistent conceptual distinctions, the aim has been to increase clarity with regard to phantasy, neurotic-belief, and other important propositional attitude types met with frequently in doing psychoa-nalysis. In this way, using a philosophical analysis the clinical theory of psychoanalysis has been provided with something of value, that is, rigor.

From the other direction, it is hoped that psychoanalytic clinical concepts about phantasy and neurotic-belief (both including unconscious content)—when properly specified—can contribute much to a general theory of mind and to the disciplines of the philosophy of mind and the philosophy of action. Currently most philosophers claim that (1) conscious and rational propositional attitudes comprise the great majority of representational mental states, and (2) that accounts of psychology featuring conscious belief/desire analyses suffice for understanding much of human behavior. Psychoanalysts know that both of those views are inadequate. In every patient, in every session, we not only assume unconscious contents and various unconscious cognitive states, we deal directly with propositional attitudes different from beliefs-proper; attitudes that are clearly contentful and yet are primary process mediated—that is, a-rational, or irrational—façades of rationality notwithstanding. It is important that we be able to communicate this knowledge beyond the consulting room and beyond our professional meetings and publications.

Chapter 8

Desire and the readiness-to-act[1]

Following Chapter 7 in which much was made of the need for a sharp distinction between the cognitive attitude types belief-proper and neurotic-belief, where neurotic-beliefs are more correctly considered as a complex of phantasy and specious reality-testing, the current chapter distinguishes between the conative attitudes desire and wish. Desires, I will claim, essentially are constituted as desires by their link to action in the real world —specifically, that the constitutive function of desire is to produce "readiness-to-act" toward fulfillment of the desire's content. Wishes, in contrast, also aim to get their content fulfilled, but do so via phantasies, not real-world actions, such that the constitutive function of wishes is to produce the right sort of phantasy.

As in Chapter 7 where important cognitive attitude confounds were presented and analyzed, in Chapter 8 we will see conative attitude confounds—in particular problems arising as desires are taken to be mere wishes. The account proposed here, distinguishing desires from wishes, when taken in conjunction with Freud's assumptions of unconscious meaningful mentation (Assumption Three) and mentation organized according to primary process as well as secondary process principles (Corollary One), helps explain the propensity to mistype. Further, in the process of more deeply understanding these conative attitude conflations, not only do the limitations of standard belief/desire views of human motivation and action lacking these psychoanalytic assumptions become obvious, but also a better account of some cases puzzling both to philosophers and psychoanalysts is provided.

Introduction

Psychological attitudes are standardly divided into two types—cognitive attitudes, in which the content of the attitude is regarded as *having come about*; and conative attitudes, in which the content *is to be brought about*. (See Velleman 2000, pp. 9–10, 11–112; See also Chapter 7, footnote 5.) When I believe *a*, that

---

[1]   I thank Timothy Schroeder and David Velleman for helpful comments on earlier versions of this chapter.

there is a water fountain 20 feet from here, from my point of view it is the case that *a*, a water fountain exists 20 feet from here. When I desire *b*, a cool drink of water, I would like *b*, my having a cool drink to be made the case. The cognitive attitude, belief, and the conative attitude, desire, are frequently paired in order to understand behavior generally and intentional action in particular. Thus, a skeletal belief/desire analysis of behavior X—the getting of a cool drink would look like this: I believe *a*, that there is a water fountain close by; I desire *b*, a cool drink; I further believe *c*, that I can bring *b* about by X-ing; and so I do X; I go to the water fountain and drink.

Beliefs are not the only cognitive attitudes—for example, for a given content *a*, that 20 feet from here is a water fountain, I can also phantasize, imagine, pretend, or suppose *a* to be the case. But belief stands apart from the other cognitive attitudes in an important way. Intrinsic to being a belief is its distinctive functional and constitutive aim in attempting to represent the world truly and correctly. If evidence to the contrary of a belief's content *a* is gained—if I am shown that what appeared to be a water fountain is really a birdbath—the belief that *a* can no long be held *as a belief*. The same negative evidence, however, in no way prevents me from continuing to phantasize *a*, imagine *a* true, pretend *a* true, or suppose *a* true. The content *a* can no longer be believed-true owing to the fact that belief functions to represent the world as it is—"belief constitutively aims at the truth" (Velleman 2000, p. 16)—and that this constitutive regulation of belief constrains what contents can be believed (as opposed to imagined, supposed, etc.).

Is a parallel constitutive aim analysis for desire, standing apart from other conative attitudes possible and useful?[2] I will argue that although such a parallel may indeed be desirable, three of the most prominent candidates for desire's constitutive aim all have fatal flaws. I will propose instead that desire has a *constitutive function*—namely, that in order to be a desire, a conative attitude must contribute to action production in the real world toward the fulfillment of its own content—a *readiness-to-act*. Wishes, I will claim, have a much different constitutive function. Wishes contribute to the fulfillment of their content, not through readiness-to-act in the real world, but via the formation of the sort of phantasies that can provide fulfillment. Later I will demonstrate that by distinguishing between the constitutive functions of desires and wishes in this way, and particularly by understanding readiness-to-act as

---

[2] A successful parallel analysis for desire would seem a positive outcome, including from the point of view of conceptual aesthetics.

desire's constitutive function, better accounts for heretofore puzzling cases can be provided. But much initial groundwork is needed.

First, I must make clear that my view of the sharp distinction between desire and wish is not widely held. To many such a distinction seems unneeded, and to some it even seems unnatural. Indeed in everyday speech "wishing" and "desiring" are often used interchangeably along with another synonym "wanting." Further, as I will elaborate in the next section both Freud and Davidson, two important figures in the realm of human action, implicitly treat wishing, desiring and wanting as interchangeable members of the same class of entities. And yet what follows immediately are two everyday examples that motivate the intuition that desires are distinct from wishes—a distinction whose nature I will later hold is based on different constitutive functional roles for wishes and desires.

Example One: I "hope" my brother, a poor student of Latin, does very well in his upcoming Latin exam, at least as well as I have and I am a great student of Latin.

On the face of it, I have introduced another conative attitude, hoping, different from wishing and desiring. But let us look more closely. There can be two distinctively different versions of my hoping, one that looks like wishing and the other desiring. In the wish-like version, although I hope he does extremely well on the Latin exam, I *do* nothing whatever to help him even though I easily could. Instead I daydream (phantasize) that he continues the family tradition of excellence in Latin. In the desire-like version, since I hope he does well, I spend hours tutoring him, teaching him as much as possible.

Example Two: Suppose that my sister has had a series of medical tests and the results are available but not yet known to me. I "hope" that the results are normal.

Again there are two versions of my hoping that her results are normal. In the wish version I can hope that the results are good—performing no actions as indeed none can influence the outcome, but imagining (phantasizing) good news. And, less rationally, with the desire version, I can hope that the results are good and accompany my hope with superstitious actions designed to bring about the unproblematic results.

While not uninteresting that "hoping" can be used in these two ways, for my purposes its importance owes to the fact that its disjunctive status reveals a fundamental distinction between desire, on the one hand, and wish on the other. My claim is that the nature of this distinction is based on the different constitutive functions of wish and desire. The first versions in each of these sample cases of hoping can be assimilated to the conative attitude of "wishing." There is no action taken toward the content of the hope/wish being fulfilled, but the hope/wish has functioned to produce phantasy material the content of which is wish-fulfilling. The second versions in each case fit as examples of "desiring." Here the contents of each desire plays the functional role of contributing a "readiness-to-act" toward its own fulfillment.

Before I present arguments for my view that wish and desire have distinct constitutive functions, I will, in the section to follow immediately, discuss three thinkers vital to this area—Freud, Davidson, Anscombe—who either make no such distinction at all, or who deem it unimportant.

Views that suggest no important distinction between wish and desire

Freud

For Freud (1905b, 1915a), each agent is at root motivated to act in the world by his/her "instinctual drives." On the border between biology and psychology and prior to any capacity for evaluative judgments, the most basic instinctual drives represent and express bodily needs and urges, whose real-world satisfaction are necessary for survival and yield pleasure much of the time. Drives seek satisfaction in a "driving," preemptory, persistent fashion, operating in accord with what Freud (1900) called the "pleasure principle."[3] Derivative and developing from this inborn biological/psychological foundation of instinctual drives (much of which is shared by higher mammals) are each person's particular, individual, strictly psychological drive instantiations. Freud called these wishes. (See Freud 1905b, 1915a; and Brenner 1982, pp. 25–6.) Wishes can be conscious or unconscious, realistic or not, acceptable or unacceptable (to the agent him/herself and those around him/her), rational or irrational,

---

[3] Despite this name and the fact that most drives are associated with pleasure, on the Freudian account it is the drive itself and not the attendant pleasure that motivates. This becomes clear with Freud's introduction of the death instinct in 1920 (*Beyond the Pleasure Principle*, SE, Vol.18, see pp. 49–57). Here drives that are accompanied by unpleasure strive for fulfillment. But even 25 years prior to that, in Freud's *Project for a Scientific Psychology* (1895) (SE, Vol. 1, pp. 281–397) he made the case that what the drive strives for is discharge operating under the "Principle of Constancy." That drives aim not only to have their content fulfilled, as is the case for all conative attitudes, but simultaneously at discharge, remains at the core of Freud's view of drives, especially with respect to what he considered the general aim of all drives. (See Chapter 6 for a discussion on the general vs. the specific aims of drives.)

trivial or momentous, satisfy-able or incapable of ever yielding satisfaction, or any permutation thereof. But no matter what their nature, particular wishes are for Freud the motivators of actions; and since the origin of even the most acceptable, realistic, and rational wish must be traced to the instinctual drives, wishes reflect their pleasure principle heritage of a driving, persistent quest for gratification.

So how are instinctual drives and wishes related to desire? Desire, unlike wish, is not a term of art for Freud; his translators did not even index this word (SE, Vol. 24 [Index]). Further, Freud addresses neither the relations nor the distinctions among wishes, hopes, wants, and desires (SE, Vol. 24 [Index]); nor have his followers, or even current-day psychoanalytic theorists. There is no listing, for example, for "desires" (or "hopes" or "wants") in the third edition of *Psychoanalytic Terms and Concepts*, published in 1990 and touted as "the popular *Glossary* of the American Psychoanalytic Association ... expanded into a mini-encyclopedia that presents both historical and current meanings of the most widely accepted psychoanalytic terms and concepts" (Excerpt from flyleaf). Looking at the German original of Freud's complete works, the words "Wunsch" (noun) and "wunchen" (verb) are used by Freud far more than any other plausible synonym (GW, Vol. 18 [Gesamtregister]) for terms Strachey (chief translator for the English Standard Edition) translates as "wish." The noun, "Wunsch," according to Langenscheidt's (1959) German/English and English/German dictionary means "wish, desire" (p. 261); and the English verbs "desire," "want," and "wish" are all translated as "wunchen" (pp. 326, 496, 500). Thus, it seems fair to conclude that insofar as he used a term in German that refers interchangeably to the English terms "wish" and "desire," for Freud particular desires no less than particular wishes developed from drives, and as such share the same driving push to be gratified.

As will be shown below, Freud's failure to differentiate wish from desire contributed to a lack of conceptual concision in aspects of psychoanalytic clinical theory. This situation can now be improved upon by making the distinction between wish and desire clear.

Davidson

Like Freud, Davidson makes no explicit distinction between wishing and desiring. Unlike Freud and his translator, Davidson uses "want," "desire," or "pro-attitude," and, rarely, "wish" to discuss conative attitudes. Thus "wish" does not appear in the index of his *Action and Events* (1980); for "wants" the reader is referred to "desires" (p. 304); while "desire" is indexed as occurring on thirteen different pages (p. 301), and "pro-attitude" appears on nine (p. 303).

Davidson (1963) states: "Wanting seems pallid beside lusting, but it would be odd to deny that someone who lusted after a woman or a cup of coffee wanted her or it. It is not unnatural, in fact, to treat wanting as a genus including all pro-attitudes as species" (p. 6).

Anscombe

For Anscombe (1957), the only conative attitude of interest is that connected with intention, and it "is neither wishing nor hoping nor the feeling of [a prick] of desire, and cannot be said to exist in a man who does nothing toward getting what he wants" (pp. 67–8). But Anscombe does begin to make a distinction between an intention-directed conative attitude and wish, a distinction I will want to make more boldly. She says:

> A chief mark of an idle wish is that a man does nothing—whether he could or no—toward the fulfillment of the wish.... The most primitive expression of wishing is e.g. "Ah, if only ...!"... I could hold the moon in the palm of my hand ... or if I were a millionaire. It is a special form of expression ... and it might be instructive to ask how such a form is identified ... but it does not concern us here." (p. 67)

Although it was not of more than passing interest to Anscombe, it is the main point of interest in this chapter. Anscombe's contrast between idle wishes and intention-directed conative attitudes, although tossed-off and rough, points the way toward the substantive distinction between wish and desire that I claim obtains—a distinction based on differences between the constitutive function of wishes such that they produce wish-fulfilling phantasy content, vs. the constitutive function of desires such that they contribute an readiness-to-act toward fulfillment of their content.

What would it be for desire to have a constitutive aim? Three (failed) proposals

In the beginning of this chapter, I indicated that finding a constitutive aim for desire, parallel to belief aiming at the truth would be desirable, although I also claimed that three prominent candidates had fatal flaws. Before getting into more detail on my proposal for desire's constitutive function, some discussion of these failed attempts for finding a constitutive aim for desire is owed.

First, what is it for a desire or any conative or cognitive attitude to have a particular constitutive aim? It consists in just three parts: (1) A constitutive aim for a cognitive or conative attitude must distinguish it from other cognitive or conative attitudes; (2) It must do so on a regulatory basis for the attitude in question, in that if an attitude does not aim in accord with the constitutive aim, it cannot be that attitude; and finally (3) The regulation must reflect a distinct functional role for the attitude in question.[4] Thus belief is distinguished from the other cognitive attitudes on the basis of its constitutively aiming at the truth. If a cognitive attitude does not so aim, it cannot be a belief (though it can remain another cognitive attitude). And aiming at the truth reflects the distinct functional role of belief (but not other cognitive attitudes) in terms of attempting to match representations of the world correctly with how the world actually is.

Anscombe's candidate

For Anscombe the constitutive aim of desire is "the good." She (1957) begins with the idea that the objects of desire possess intrinsic desirability characteristics, that is, they are good in some fashion (p. 70). Her account of the good evolves, however, and soon (p. 76) she asserts that what is desired is that which is subjectively regarded as good by the agent, which may not be "what is really good." Nonetheless, Anscombe is able to maintain that there is a parallel between judgment (belief) aiming for truth, and wanting (desire) aiming for good: "Truth is the object of judgment, and good the object of wanting; it does not follow from this either that everything judged must be true, or that everything wanted must be good" (p. 76).

This seems right as far as it goes, and yet a vital aspect of the parallel does not hold. If I *believe* X and then I am *shown* that X is not true, I can no longer *believe* X. I can phantasize X, I can pretend X is true, but I can no longer *believe* X. But if I *desire* Y, not only can I be *shown* that Y is not good and still *desire* Y, I myself can regard Y as not good, and continue to *desire* Y. I can have perverse desires ranging from the truly sadistic to those entailing various forms of self-destruction, all the while knowing for myself subjectively that the objects of these desires are not good. I can, nevertheless, continue to *desire* this not-good object; the status of the desire as-a-desire unchanged. Thus, on the grounds that it cannot regulate membership as a desire sufficiently (condition 2 above), Anscombe's candidate for desire's constitutive aim—the good—does not hold up.

---

[4] Readiness-to-act as desire's constitutive function does distinguish desire from other conative attitudes, and this is the case in virtue of its distinct functional role, but there is no regulatory aim. In other words, a desire aims to get its content fulfilled and it *does this via action-readiness*; but a desire *does not aim to fulfill its aim via action*.

Davidson's candidate

For Donald Davidson (1978), to desire something is to regard it as desirable—"the desirable" is desire's constitutive aim. This is more complex then it sounds. To desire something if it is desirable entails aiming for something over and above the *to-be-brought-about* aim intrinsic to desire and to every conative attitude. What Davidson adds is this: in my desiring that X be brought about, I have also *judged* X and the state of its being brought about as desirable, *worthy of desire*. As Velleman (2000, p. 116) puts it "Davidson's [1978] claim that to desire something is to regard it as desirable … seems to say that to desire something is to have an attitude toward it as worthy of that very attitude."

Davidson's view is not without appeal. First, although he himself did not make this claim, his view of desire's constitutive aim allows desire to be singled out from other conative attitudes in the same way belief can stand apart from other cognitive attitudes. So a Davidsonian could claim that when someone wishes or hopes for X although he/she regards it as something to be brought about, unlike the case for desire, there is no entailed commitment that he/she finds X itself or the state of its being brought about as something desirable, something that ought to be brought about. Thus on Davidson's view, moreso than on Anscombe's, there could be a parallel between the constitutive aims of belief and desire: Just as to believe Y true implies that Y ought really be true; to desire X be brought about implies that X is something really worthy of being brought about.

But there is a serious problem. Not only are Davidson's candidates for the constitutive aim for belief and desire parallel, they both are regulated by evaluative judgments or correctness—something appropriate only to belief[5] and not intrinsic to desire. Velleman (2000, pp. 116–17) sums up the trouble:

> The claim that to desire something is to regard it as desirable is … not just that the propositional object of desire is regarded as something to be made true or brought about, but also that it is so regarded with the aim of getting things right …[and] … nothing about desire entitles us to credit it with the justificatory force of a value judgment.

---

[5] Stampe (1987, pp. 355–6) in fact raises the point that this sort of judgment of worthiness—in his words (and his emphasis) —"*its being good that it be the case that p*," does not sufficiently distinguish desires from some beliefs. Using the example of a new job that one believes it would be good to take, Stampe claims that one need not have any desire to take it. Indeed one need not have such a desire; but this is no challenge to Davidson's view of desire. In assessing the job as something it would be good to take, only the additional 'judging as worthy of being brought about' aspect of Davidsonian desire is present, not the necessary initial pro-attitude, that from the agent's view the new job is something *to be brought about*.

Even Davidson (1963) in admitting that "a man may have a yen, say, to drink a can of paint, without ever, even at the moment he yields, believing it would be worth doing" (p. 4) provides an example that must count against his own view that desire aims constitutively toward desirability.[6]

Velleman's candidate

Velleman (2000) has an alternative candidate for desire's constitutive aim, but he states at the outset that it is not a parallel with the constitutive aim for belief. In his view no good parallel exists. "When we consider how desire differs in aim from other modes of conation, we find that the difference is not analogous to that between belief and other modes of cognition" (p. 116). He continues, "The difference in aim between desire and other conative attitudes appears to be that desire aims, not at the good, but rather at the attainable (p. 116) … desire has the attainable as its constitutive aim" (p. 117). He explains that although one can wish for something even when its truth seems impossible and hope for something even when it is already the case, "one can desire that p only if p seems attainable, in the sense of being a possible future outcome" (pp. 116–17).

This candidate for desire's constitutive aim not only lacks what would be the aesthetically pleasing conceptual parallel with belief's constitutive aim, but also has three additional problems.

First, and somewhat trivial, since determining what is attainable is frequently difficult, the ascription of the proper conative attitude type would often be post-hoc.

Second and more important, it is not clear that Velleman's constitutive aim accurately picks out desire from among other conative attitudes. Thus it fails on condition 1 for constituting a constitutive aim (see pp. 140–141 above), and here is how it fails. Bratman (1999, pp. 19–20, 32, 121) in arguing for intending as a distinct mental state not reducible to an agent's beliefs and desires, discusses conflicting desires. Suppose I both want to go to the movies now and finish working on this section of this chapter now. These are each attainable alone, but they are not both attainable together. With Velleman's constitutive aim for desire one must conclude that although each of them is a desire when alone, they both are not desires when they occur simultaneously. Bratman (p. 32), however, points out that this sort of conflict between desires is routine and that "we do not normally require our desires to be consistent in these ways."

---

[6] This assumes that to "have a yen" is synonymous with to "have a desire," a reading that is certainly suggested by the context.

Instead it is our plans or *intentions* that have to be attainable: "If ... my *plans include* both actions then I *am* guilty of a criticizable form of inconsistency" (p. 32). Attainability, then, is putatively a more fitting constitutive aim for intentions.

The third problem for Velleman's candidate for desire's constitutive aim is that attainability does not seem to regulate desire very adequately. It is just as plausible and natural to desire *p*, as to wish or hope for *p* even if *p* is unattainable. There are at least two types of such cases. First, there are very unrealistic desires. Z has an unloving parent. No matter what he has done to try to please her over his entire 50 years, she has remained cold. Although he knows this full well, he unrealistically desires her love and continues to act so as to attempt to gain it. He does so even knowing that his desire is unrealistic. Then, the second type of cases involves actually impossible desires. My desire to live forever (sadly) falls into this class. But I do desire immortality, and I act in every way I can to make my living forever the case, even though I know full well there is no way whatever for me to be successful.

The constitutive function of desire and the constitutive function of wish

As each of the above accounts of constitutive aim for desire has failed, I will propose, instead that desire has a *constitutive function*—namely, that in order to be a desire, a conative attitude must contribute to action production in the real world toward the fulfillment of its own content—a *readiness-to-act*. Wishes, I will claim, have a much different constitutive function. Wishes contribute to the fulfillment of their content, not through readiness-to-act in the real world, but via the formation of the sort of phantasies that can provide fulfillment. I will argue for this view in three ways. First, that several potentially damaging problems to this view can be overcome. Next, that various counterexamples can also be handled. Third, that with the proposed constitutive function for wish and especially that for desire in place certain puzzling cases can be better understood.

Potential problems for readiness-to-act as desire's constitutive function

Fanciful desires and realistic wishes

The unrealistic desire for love from an unloving parent and the impossible desire for immortality are not problematic for a view in which desire has as its constitutive function a readiness-to-act in the real world toward its own fulfillment. Z continues to *act* to please his mother in order to gain her love, and I continue to perform *actions* designed to endlessly prolong my life, even though Z is aware of his unrealistic desire, and I of my impossible one. It is the real world activity toward the fulfillment of the content of these conative attitudes that marks them as *desires*, notwithstanding the contents' unrealistic or impossible nature. In contrast, wishes on my account produce wish-fulfilling phantasies and do not lead to readiness-to-act. Although one perhaps could hold that this is due to the sometimes fanciful content of wishes, I propose instead that it owes to the formal structure of wishes. After all, just as some desires can be impossible, some wishes can be anything but fanciful. I, for example, wish George W. Bush was not and had never been President; and although this is a strong and realistic wish, it is a wish. I have phantasies that my wish is fulfilled; but I will not act on it in any way.[7]

Strong wishes and weak desires

But do strong wishes and weak desires pose trouble for my view? Do strong wishes demonstrate readiness-to-act, while weak desires do not? It seems implausible to contend that increased wish strength could produce increased activity of the relevant sort. Think of wishing mildly vs. wishing fervently for Bush to no longer be President. I do in fact hold this wish strongly, but I still will not act on ending his presidency prematurely.

But the weak desire claim is more serious. I have two possible moves. I could assert that weak desires are indeed desires no less, despite reduced readiness-to-act, claiming that if a "weak desire" actually motivated *no* impetus toward its fulfillment, it would really not be a desire at all, just an "idle" wish. Otherwise, as long as it occasions some such impetus, it is properly considered a "desire." Or, I could claim that weak desires are structurally quite like strong desires in terms of action potential, but other factors intervene (including e.g. conflicting desires) such that a weakened desire results.[8] Both positions describe phenomena that obtain and I will avail myself of both. What is not tenable is holding that "weak desires" *are* just "wishes" for it is essential to my view that desires, weak and strong, have the same constitutive function. Thus, any desire functions constitutively to produce (or to contribute to the production) of readiness-to-act toward the real-world fulfillment of its own content—far

---

[7] One might argue that no action is possible for me. While that is true regarding his never having been President, actions are possible about his being President. I could write to my Congressional representatives and urge impeachment and removal. And, if I were a very unbalanced person I might act so as to attempt to physically harm or even kill him.

[8] The quantitative effects produced by conflicting desires will be discussed later in this section.

different from any wish whose constitutive function is the production of phantasies (not real-world actions) of the sort that can provide wish-fulfillment, (not real-world satisfaction).

Intending

The matter of intending raises another potential difficulty. Does intending also function to produce something very much like a readiness-to-act? If so how does my claim for readiness-to-act as *desire's constitutive function* hold up? A closer look reveals that intending and desiring do not have the same constitutive functions, as it is clear that the regulations on intending are less demanding. Intending requires (and functionally produces) only a conditional readiness-to-act, a readiness-to-act projected sometime into the future. Thus, whenever I at time t, intend to do X at time $t+2$, it is implied that my intention *now* is do X at time $t+2$, *unless* at some time between *now* and $t+2$ I change my mind. On the other hand, when I desire to do X, my readiness-to-act is *now*; I am "action-ready" in the service of the desire.[9] Desiring and intending are separate conative attitudes with different constitutive functions.

Future desires

The discussion on intending, referring to future actions, leads to the consideration of another potential problem: Can my view of desire's constitutive function account for future desires?[10] Take for example my "desire" to visit Australia sometime, my husband's "desire" to write a book on the Portuguese language when he retires, and our "desire" to get another dog when we have sufficiently mourned the death of our last one. What if in each of these cases there is no obvious present tense readiness-to-act, not even on the level of thought-activity about relevant actions preceding real-world actions? Does this mean that on my view these are not desires? That is certainly a possibility, but not a conclusion I will draw without the further investigation, which follows directly.

---

[9] Along with the constitutive function differences, there is also another important factor differentiating these two conative attitudes. As discussed above, intending but not desiring must be regulated by what is regarded as attainable. This includes the fact that while desires can conflict, intentions must be consistent.

[10] The anonymous referee to whom I owe the discussion of this topic, suggested that desires of long-standing might also present difficulties for my view. But insofar as there is a present element to any long-standing desire, readiness-to-act as the constitutive function is unproblematic.

In claiming to have a desire about the future, at least one of two mental operations involving time seem natural and required. One is imagining that future conditions obtain now. The other is projecting one's current conative attitude into the future. Suppose that I desire to visit Australia but cannot get away this year. Now (time t) I imagine that it is some later time ($t + 2$) when such a trip is feasible. If under these conditions I feel that I would indeed still desire to go to Australia, I could plausibly hold that I have a future desire to go to Australia. The other sort of operation, conative attitude projection, is slightly different but related. Now (at time t) I desire to go to Australia, but I cannot. Again, I think about a future time ($t + 2$) when I can go to Australia. To the extent that I can truly make the following statement—"if I feel then as I do now, then I will desire to go to Australia"—I have projected my current desire for this trip into the future, and I plausibly have a future desire to go to Australia. But are all of these putative "future desires" actual desires? Again, what about those seemingly without readiness-to-act?

Let me first say that many such putative "future desires" can, on my account, be considered actual desires without any problem, given *any* sort of readiness-to-act now (at time t). For example, if I were to be seeking information now about Australia, or about my vacation schedule at $t + 2$. Further, my view has no problem handling conative attitudes that change as time $t + 2$ approaches. My husband now (time t) has a desire to write his book at $t + 2$ and he is currently assembling his old articles and other references. But what if at $t + 1$ he no longer wants to do it? His conative attitude at time t was still a desire, not a wish regardless of his attitude at $t + 1$ and $t + 2$.

However, there is a class of putative future desires without any obvious readiness-to-act now (at time t) that is admittedly much more problematic for my view. This sort of "future" desire would occasion no present-day activity related to its fulfillment, no obvious readiness-to-act, even at the level of relevant thought-activity, and so on my view, would not properly qualify as a desire. And yet in such cases the agent in question might well, in performing one or both of the mental temporal operations described just above, claim to have a "future desire." How can I contend that such agential assertion is insufficient?

I do so advancing the view that desiring as a conative mental attitude is not transparent. Agents do not have consistent privileged access as to whether, using my terms, they desire rather than wish for something even in the present. In fact, as I will take up at length below in the section on "Miscategorizing conative attitudes" there is often a confounding of these two conative attitude types. Certainly then, conative attitudes about the future have no immunity to this sort of miscategorizing and may even be more vulnerable. And yet, it is hard to conclude the sort of agent-embraced "future desire" now under consideration is always a mere wish. It may be that this sort of future directed conative attitude is some inchoate combination of wish and desire, much as is true of the conative attitudes of very young children (see below), with the differentiation between these two attitudes to emerge only as time unfolds.

Summarizing, readiness-to-act as desire's constitutive function affords only moderate success in dealing adequately with future desires. On the positive side (1) many "future desires" qualify as desires with no difficulty; (2) there is no problem for future desires that change as time progresses; and (3) owing to no consistent privileged access and no transparency, some conative attitudes regarded as future desires are not desires, just as some present tense conative attitudes are miscategorized. However on the negative side (1) a certain type of plausible "future desire"—embraced by the agent as a desire but without readiness-to-act—admits of a conative attitude categorization that is at best vague. On my account such future desires cannot properly be categorized as desires and yet it is not at all clear that they are mere wishes. Some combination, not unlike that seen in early childhood might best describe these states.

Conflicting desires

Are conflicting desires a problem for positing readiness-to-act as the constitutive function of desire? Above I held that while it is expected that intentions be attainable, and thereby consistent with one another and not conflicting, there is no such stricture on desires. Desires can be mutually exclusive and yet each can manifest a readiness-to-act. The desire with the greater readiness-to-act is, *ceteris paribus*, the one satisfied. This sort of "psychological calculus" is performed quite automatically much of the time. Take a simple case. Suppose I have two free hours this Friday afternoon and that I have three desires, one is to take a bicycle ride, the second is to get started on some household errands, and the third is to make some progress on this chapter. Many rather subtle activities manifest my readiness-to-act on each of these. I note that the weather is perfect for bike riding and that I do have my helmet with me. I make a list (physical or mental) of the errands that are necessary for the weekend. And I think about the issues in this chapter reviewing internally where I left off. Then I begin to work on the chapter and write. The readiness-to-act for this desire, now this Friday afternoon, is greater than that for the other two actions, either of which I was also capable of performing.

Mature vs. immature desires demonstrate another type of conflict between desires. Suppose that a friend and I are playing racquetball and that I am inadvertently hit. I have a visceral desire to retaliate by inflicting pain and I feel my body lunging in that direction. Realizing I have been hurt accidentally, I also have a desire to be civilized. Hence I move (actually, countermove or brake) so as to override and inhibit the retributive action, such that my more mature desire wins out (usually).

A more complicated situation with conflicted desires is due to my husband (who was trying to come up with a case my view could not explain). He remembered that when he went to high school dances he noticed that one unusually pretty girl, G, was always surrounded by a number of average-looking female friends, A–F. The average girls liked G, probably for a number of reasons, but one was that the boys were so attracted to pretty G that they would inexorably move toward her and thereby toward all of them. This eventuated in girls A–F actually getting asked to dance more often than G! According to my husband the boys desired G more, and yet they more often asked the average girls to dance. How could my psychological calculus concerning quantitative degrees of readiness-to-act account for the fact that while the boys demonstrated their readiness-to-act by moving toward the pretty girl they desired most (desire G), they chose partners they seemed to desire less (desire A or B or C ... F etc.)? The puzzle is solved once we realized that there was another desire here, one uppermost for a great many adolescent boys, the desire to not feel humiliated by the pretty girl saying "no thanks." (Let us call this desire H). Using the psychological calculus, although desire G has more readiness-to-act than desire A (or B ... etc.), desire H has more than desire G. Once this is understood, fulfilling desire H plus desire A (or B ... etc.) seems like a good deal.

Related to these cases are conflicted desires seen in neuroses, in which what is desired is regarded as unacceptable and therefore to be defended against. Variations of this type of conflict will be taken up at length in the section on "Puzzling cases" below, but here is a brief example specifically involving desires used to defend against other desires. Richard desires to complete his Ph.D. He is having a lot of trouble finishing, but he keeps trying. When he talks about his difficulty, it becomes increasingly clear that he neurotically (and unconsciously) equates getting a Ph.D. with outdoing and actually defeating his father, something he (unconsciously) desires but finds unacceptable and desires to inhibit. So on one side of the readiness-to-act equation is Richard's desire for his Ph.D. plus his (unconscious) desire to defeat his dad. On the other side is his (unconscious) desire to override the activity which will bring about the (unconsciously) desired, but unacceptable harm to his father. It is unclear which side will prevail.

Finally, there are conflicting desires that are handled sequentially. First there are simple examples of this. I want to spend a quiet evening at home with my family, but I also want to go to my colleague's weekly party. Although these desires are mutually exclusive at a particular time, there is little problem with spending some time at home and then coming to the party later. Or I can decide to stay at home this week and go to the party next week.

Frequently, however, these matters are more difficult. I can be with a patient and judge that two sorts of interpretative comments might further the analysis. One concerns the patient's past history and the other is about his/her feeling in the analysis now—the transference. Each comment would likely stimulate a whole different set of associations, each quite important. I desire to make both now. But I must make only one and wait for some propitious time to make the other. In experimental work as well, a researcher can desire to test a certain hypothesis with not one but two experiments, each with a design equally feasible and as likely to adequately test the hypothesis at stake. If one's resources are limited one must choose one, and based on the results do the other as a follow-up.

A more complex type of sequential handling of conflicted desires can be found in child development. Children desire immediate gratification of several sorts. They not only want to eat when and what they want, they want to urinate and defecate when and wherever they feel the urge. Further, children often desire to go wherever they want without restriction. On top of all of this they want to express their frustration in immediate, unmodulated, physical ways. But these ubiquitous desires are in conflict with a profound desire every child has to please his/her parents. How does this dilemma get resolved? Certainly not in the same fashion as the simpler sequential cases above: children cannot please their parents at one time and then sometime later gratify all desires immediately. No, the key seems to be that through the overarching desire to please parents, the child learns that he/she can indeed eat, drink, defecate, urinate, in fact satisfy many other desires but only in a specified structured way—a *sequential* way which is learned over a great deal of time. A child learns he/she can and should defecate, but not now and especially not here—one must wait until one is at a toilet. And a child learns he/she can eat chocolate, just not now before dinner.

Perhaps the most interesting and problematic sort of sequentially acted upon conflicted desires are seen in akrasia. The akratic has two mutually exclusive desires, for example to diet, restricting calories, and at the same time to eat fattening foods. And, while he/she judges the dieting to be the better act, he/she eats fattening foods. But a more fine-grained look at this reveals that akratics are actually sequentially satisfying one desire and then another. Take Mr O who would like to lose 50 pounds and be at a weight that he once maintained. He realizes this would not only be good for his health, but he would look and feel better. Let us (arbitrarily) say the sequence began with Mr O gratifying his desire for fattening foods such that he had a 50-pound weight gain. Then as he embarked and stayed on a diet, his desire for restricting calories and losing weight was the desire upon which he acted. But later when his resolve dissolved and he was again overeating, the desire for fattening foods prevailed. This sequential pattern can be observed in most akratics. The smoker who wants to quit, smokes his/her "last" cigarette (acting on the desire to smoke), and until his/her next cigarette (which represents the lapse) is actively not smoking (acting on the desire to quit). Perhaps akratics would meet with more success if their conflicting desires were experienced differently. Suppose instead of the conflicting desires consisting in smoking this cigarette (desire A) vs. not smoking this cigarette (desire B) at particular time t, the conflicting desires experienced were, being a smoker (desire A') vs. being a nonsmoker (desire B'), and not just at time t, but also at $t + 1$, $t + n$ ..., in other words in general. This reconfiguring would render impossible the typical akratic's sequential but viciously circular way of dealing with his/her conflicting desires.[11] (There is more on akrasia below in the section on "Puzzling cases.")

Counterexamples to the proposed constitutive function for desire

Can the proposed constitutive function for desires hold up when faced with three sorts of potentially problematic counterexamples? First, there are tics and habits. Tics, commonly defined as repeated, abnormal, impulsive muscular movements or vocalizations, manifest an action-readiness. But as is clear from both Anscombe (1957) and Davidson (1963), it is important to differentiate truly intentional actions from other sorts of actions, for example, mere motor behaviors, whereby only the truly intentional acts are caused in the right way by desire (and belief). Tics, then although behavioral actions, are not acts associated with any conative attitude, where a conative attitude is by definition directed toward "making some content the case that." Thus, tics do no damage to the constitutive function of desire proposed here, for tics do not count as the sort of actions produced by desires and their constitutive readiness-to-act function.

Let us turn now to habits, including both innocuous ones like always choosing the same complex route from Point A to Point B, and less benign habits like nail biting and various compulsive actions. Different from tics, all sorts of habits do clearly demonstrate an agent's readiness-to-act in order to bring about the habit's content. Compulsive actions and habits therefore, not

---

[11] How to effect this sort of reconfiguring is a baffling clinical problem outside the scope of this book.

withstanding the fact that an agent will often report that these actions are performed automatically, unconsciously, or even involuntarily, on my account *do* actually demonstrate the agent's readiness-to-act following from a desire. (Compulsive actions in particular will be discussed further in the section on "Puzzling cases" below.)

Second, there is another class of potential counterexample—attitudes that some may classify as desires despite no manifestation of readiness-to-act. These are exemplified by cases in which Y is putatively desired, but the agent takes no action toward gaining Y even though such actions are available for the agent. For example, my mother for years claimed that she wanted to make more money. Although there were many things she could have done to increase her earnings, and she phantasized rather happily about each of them, she never did a thing to change her money-making mechanisms. On my account attitudes such as these should not be considered desires at all. They are wishes, producing wish-fulfilling phantasies, not desire-producing real-world actions; they are wishes miscategorized as desires. Now admittedly I have made no argument. I have shaped my claim for classifying this sort of conative attitude already presuming wish-fulfilling phantasy as the constitutive function of wishes and readiness-to-act as the constitutive function of desires. And yet reasons to classify such phantasy-rich, action-less conative attitudes as desires seem equally arbitrary, without the gain in conceptual clarity.

Third and perhaps most problematic for my view is a type of desire that on the face of it seems far removed from the realm of action and readiness-to-act. I allude here to the sorts of second-order desires that Frankfurt discusses (1988, especially p. 16) in which a person desires to change the nature of his/her desire. Can Frankfurt have intended that these sorts of second-order desires have a relation to action that is more than just metaphoric? Can these second-order desires be assimilated to the view that desires constitutively function to produce a readiness-to-act toward their own fulfillment? Surprisingly, the interpretation of Frankfurt given by Dennett (1981) helps my case. Dennett states, "As Frankfurt points out, second-order desires are an empty notion unless one can act on them … Acting on a second-order desire, doing something to bring it about … is acting upon oneself" (p. 284).

In the next several sections the proposed candidate for desire's constitutive function will be shown to have two important advantages. These have to do with the explanatory power gained in two interrelated domains when readiness-to-act is taken as desire's constitutive function. The two domains involve (1) clarification of certain aspects of psychoanalytic theory, and (2) explanations of puzzling cases, puzzling both to philosophers of mind and action and to psychoanalysts. But before we move to these sections, there remains one further matter to consider. In Chapter 7 (see also Brakel 2001), I discussed a frequently occurring confound between two cognitive attitudes; specifically that phantasies are (mis)taken for beliefs. I noted that often these conflations have deleterious consequences, and proposed that this owed to the privileged role belief has with respect to action. In the section below, I will suggest that people can likewise confound wishes and desires. This too has troubling results, because desire, with readiness-to-act as its constitutive function, also has a privileged role with respect to action.[12]

Miscategorizing conative attitudes

Belief is the cognitive attitude that aims at the truth. If one gets convincing evidence that X does not obtain, one cannot continue to believe X-true. One can continue to phantasize X, imagine X-true, hypothesize-X true, but one can no longer believe X-true. Nonetheless it is a commonplace of psychoanalytic practice that patients have persistent conscious "beliefs" they know are not true. As we saw in Chapter 7, one patient "believes" that he is of no importance to his friends, family, and analyst, despite clear daily demonstrations to the contrary. Another patient "believes" she can prevent sexual attacks she suffered 60 years ago as a young child by being unengaged with men now, even though she knows that present actions cannot effect changes in the past. And these cases are not at all unusual. So what is going on? I have proposed in Chapter 7 (and Brakel 2001) that the propositional attitude in question is not a belief at all—but instead closer to another cognitive attitude—a phantasy, usually a fairly complex phantasy. "Neurotic-beliefs," like all phantasies, and unlike beliefs, do not have aiming at the truth or correctness of their content as their constitutive aim. But here is the problem: although the cognitive attitude *is* a phantasy, in some important ways it *is experienced and treated* as a belief, playing the same causal functional role belief plays with respect to action. This has significant and deleterious consequences, precisely because beliefs function centrally in the causing, explaining, and initiating actions.

---

[12] Note that although both belief and desire have privileged access to action, this privilege owes to quite different sources. This is not surprising since belief and desire have very different intrinsic natures. As beliefs are regulated by their contents being true or correct, it is prudent to predicate actions based on these accurate world-to-mind representations. Desires, on the other hand, with their origin in the instinctual drives—biologically based forces, preemptory and relentless—have a readiness-to-act (about which I am making the further claim that it is desire's constitutive function). Agents with such action-ready desires (as opposed say to wishes or hopes) are ready to act, prudent or not, toward actually bringing about in fact the mind-to-world content of their desires.

Thus, the woman with the "neurotic-belief" that she can change her past experience of abuse by her current behavior, *acts* intentionally so as to keep any and all males far away.[13]

Does a similar miscategorization, with wish mistaken for action-linked desire, occur for conative attitudes? I suggest that miscategorizations do frequently take place, but often in the opposite direction—desire being miscategorized as wish. But before that can be demonstrated, I must make clear in what ways my position on wishes and desires follows Freud's and where it differs.

Recall the discussion earlier in this chapter showing that Freud, and psychoanalysts thereafter, have not formally distinguished "desire" and "wish" from one another as distinct pro-attitudes. Thus for Freud it follows naturally that all wishes/desires are considered psychological instantiations of the biologically rooted instinctual drives. On my view too, wishes *and* desires do both derive from the drives. But they are different, with desires remaining far closer to the action orientation of the instinctual drive. This may seem controversial to psychoanalysts, and so I owe a thorough explanation.

Let me start with the fact that Freud's translators (and thereby English-speaking psychoanalysts) translated Freud's "Wunsch" as "wish" much more often than they translated it as "desire," particularly when referring to the pro-attitudes of children and the infantile (often unconscious) pro-attitudes of adults. But that particular translation choice is not the real problem. What is problematic is that Freud did not recognize these early infantile pro-attitudes as some sort of conglomerate of wish and desire. And there are several reasons to do so. Consider first that young children, much as they cannot yet separate phantasy from belief, likewise cannot distinguish between wishes and desires. For the very young every pro-attitude is linked to striving for gratification in every way possible, through both action and phantasy. Then there are two developmental matters, (1) the fact that very young children are far less effective than adults in *bringing about* anything through their own actions, so that most real-world satisfactions require parental actions, and (2) it is likely the case that for very young children a sharp differentiation between real-world satisfaction and phantasy gratification may not yet be in place.

---

[13] Although outside the scope of this chapter, the understanding that "neurotic-beliefs" are subjectively felt to be beliefs and therefore acted upon as beliefs, whereas really they are closer in attitude type to phantasies, provides a useful explanation as to why cognitive behavioral therapy (CBT) is often disappointing. CBT can help a person right a false belief or even a set of them, but it is quite ineffective in changing these long-standing central phantasy-laden neurotic-beliefs. (See Chapter 7.)

But, as he did not appreciate that in the very early life of humans there exist mostly such conglomerated wish/desire conative attitudes, Freud did not take into account developmental advances in the conative attitudes—something he was very able to do with the cognitive attitudes. In other words, while central to Freud's overall contribution is an understanding of the developing capacity to distinguish the cognitive attitude of reality-tested belief from that of phantasy, Freud's conceptual conflation of desire and wish precludes a parallel psycho-analytic understanding of the development of conative attitude maturation, which includes making the distinction between wish and desire.

Indeed for adult agents there is a significant difference between desires that one will act on to carry out, and wishes about which one muses and fulfills in phantasy. And yet adult agents frequently treat (and/or attempt to treat) action-linked desires as mere wishes. This has untoward consequences far beyond the simple conflation of terms "wish" and "desire." Since wishes and the wish-fulfilling phantasies they produce occasion no serious harm, it follows that agents might try to avoid responsibility for various unacceptable and forbidden desires, and the readiness-to-act that they produce, by mistaking these desires for wishes. However, given the persistent, insistent, drive-based nature of desires, attempting to regard and treat them as innocuous and action-distant wishes can be but a temporizing measure, with an agent's defenses against his/her hidden unconscious desires often quite self-damaging. Case 3 and in a more complicated fashion Case 4 below are examples of this sort of miscategorization. First though, from an expository point of view, there is a simpler class of miscategorizations. In Cases 1 and 2 it is the interpreters of the cases, rather than the agents themselves, who miscategorize desires as wishes. I turn to these now.

Puzzling cases

Case 1: Goethe and his baby brother

Freud (1917, pp. 145–56) read of one Goethe's early memories. The event took place at around the time Goethe's younger brother was born. The future writer hurled crockery out a window and watched it crash to the ground. Freud connected it with a report from one of *his* patients who had a memory of a similar activity. The patient remembered that his episode of plate throwing occurred around the same time he attempted murderous attacks on his baby brother. Freud hypothesized that like his patient, Goethe wished to be rid of his younger sibling and further hypothesized that throwing the plates out the window was a "symbolic or … *magic* action" (1917, p. 152) version of throwing his brother out. (This case is discussed in Velleman 2000, pp. 267–8, and 268–9, n. 49.)

Here is a standard psychoanalytic account: Goethe had a wish (conative attitude) to be rid of his baby brother and a phantasy (cognitive attitude) of throwing him out the window. This phantasy presents the wish as fulfilled. Then he acted (throwing the crockery standing for his brother) out the window. This act had a motive (wish to be rid of brother), and if we follow Freud, the reason and cause for this "magic action" was that throwing the crockery out the window would in some way fulfill that wish.

Freud's basic understanding of this case seems sound. Goethe's act of hurling the brother-representing crockery out the window was motivated by Goethe's conative attitude, which has the content "it should be made the case that we get rid of this intruder and so I throw the baby out the window." Velleman (2000, pp. 267–9, 269, n. 49), along the same lines elaborates, "What leads the child to phantasize that he is throwing out the baby is … that he wishes to *do* it" (p. 268). But then Velleman follows with a most incisive question. After noting that various philosophers (Wohlheim 1979 and Gardner 1993, both cited in Velleman 2000, p. 268, n. 48), "conceive of phantasy as shorting the motivational circuit that connects conation with outward behavior," Velleman asks, "Why does young Goethe actually throw crockery out of the window, if his wish can be gratified internally, by phantasies of expelling his younger sibling?" (p. 269, n.48). With the account proposed here for readiness-to-act as desire's constitutive function, I can now answer this excellent question. Goethe's actual pitching of the crockery (standing for the younger brother) and smashing it to the ground was motivated not by a *wish* to be rid of his baby sibling; but by his *desire* to actually throw his brother out the window—to actually *do* it. And for desire, there is no way to short-circuit action. Quite to the contrary, the constitutive function of desire is to be ready to *act*.

Only with a person's later developmental sophistication would we expect the capacity to routinely relegate unacceptable desires—such as that of an older brother to dispose of his baby brother—to the realm of wishes, where phantasies alone can gratify.[14] That phantasies, clearly not attitudes regulated by the truth, can as such gratify wishes, at least some of the time, is part of their

---

[14] This is not to say that such gratification in symbolic action does not also occur in adults. (See Hursthouse 1991 for some adult examples.) In adults however, developmental gains have made another route available: unacceptable desires can be transformed into wishes, harmless because they can be gratified without action, through phantasy alone.

biological proper function. (See Chapter 5 and Brakel 2002 for a much fuller analysis of the proper function of phantasies.)[15]

Case 2: Two desires, not two wishes

The next case concerns one of Freud's patients (1907, pp. 120–2; Velleman 2000, also discusses this example, pp. 267, 268). Here, a standard psychoanalytic view miscasts two important desires as wishes. The patient meanwhile experiences just one desire, but a desire whose content is both trivial and bizarre. Freud (1907, p. 121) discusses his patient's symptoms: "Over a period of time she used to repeat an especially noticeable and senseless action. She would run out of her room into another room in the middle of which was a table. She would straighten the tablecloth on it in a particular manner and ring for the housemaid. The latter had to come up to the table, and the patient would then dismiss her on some indifferent errand." Freud continues "at one place on the table-cloth there was a stain, and she always arranged the cloth in such a way that the housemaid was bound to see the stain." At some point Freud and the patient could piece together that this symptom was a thinly disguised repetition of events during and just after her troubled wedding night. Her husband had been impotent, but kept trying to penetrate her, running from his room to hers. The next day the new husband, concerned about the housemaid's opinion of him, took red ink to the sheets. But he did a bad job of this too.

The standard psychoanalytic account holds that this woman is reenacting the wedding night with the first wish being that her husband had not been impotent, that is, that he could have put the red stain in the right place for the right reason. This wish is of course impossible to fulfill.

---

[15] For a neuroscientifically grounded account of how wishes can be gratified internally, that is, by phantasy, see Schroeder (2004). Although Schroeder does not use the terms "wish" or "phantasy," his reward theory of desire provides a very plausible mechanism for such internal gratification. Noting that for Schroeder there is no important distinction between desire and wish (pp. 132, 166); he holds that to desire or wish something is to represent that something as constituting a reward to oneself. To do this requires that the representational capacities of the sensory and association cortex and the hypothalamus be connected to structures of the "reward system—the ventral tegmental area (VTA) and the pars compacta of the substantia nigra (SNpc). In the reward system incoming representations (i.e. contents of desires and wishes, etc.) are compared with representations of expected reward (pp. 49–50). Note that there are no requirements about the accuracy of the representations. Thus a wish can be *represented as* fulfilled—constituting a phantasy and, more important, constituting a reward which as such can '…drive the production of a reward … signal" (p. 134); and thereby gratify without action.

To understand the second wish, Velleman, thinking psychoanalytically, looks at other facts of the case—that for a time she left her husband, that she contemplated other marriage partners, and that she finally did settle on staying with her husband. Thus at the time of the acts with the stain and the maid, Velleman concludes that she wished to leave her husband, but suggests that she felt she could only do so if her leaving would not impugn his masculine prowess. The stain shown to the housemaid then "proves" that her husband now has no potency problem (2000, p. 267). This second wish, the wish to leave her husband, is unacceptable or at least ambivalently held.

Continuing with the standard account, the usual claim is that she performs the actions with the stain and the housemaid, owing to these two wishes—these wishes are the cause. And that the actions are, like Goethe's throwing of crockery, enactments of a phantasy of her wishes fulfilled—he was potent then, and he is potent now so I can leave him.

But I contend that this patient's action was caused by two desires, not wishes, just as Goethe's crockery throwing action was caused by a desire to throw his brother out, not merely a wish. First, as with Goethe's case, there is the behavior in the real world suggesting desire, with its strong link to action, as the causative conative attitude. But here there is also the repetitive nature of the woman's symptomatic phantasy action. Does the repetitiveness lend support to wishes or desires as the underlying problem?

Let us take the first conative attitude: she wishes or desires that her husband would have been potent and done the stain right on the wedding night. If this were a wish, there would be the possibility of gratification in a phantasy, and/or recognizing it as just a wish, with no need to *do* anything toward its fulfillment. As a desire, it is of course an impossible desire that can never be fulfilled. Thus proposing that Freud's patient suffered from an impossible desire explains better her repetitive *readiness-to-act* toward its fulfillment, rather than to assign its content—that her husband would have been potent and performed marital intercourse well on their wedding night—to the category of wish, mere wish, the real world fulfillment of which would not be sought.[16]

---

[16] Given the forgoing, is it possible that many neurotic repetitive actions have the same underlying impossible desire-driven rather than wish-driven causes? A look at the other puzzling cases below lends some support to this idea. Note however that this is not to say that there are not other causes of repeated actions. In fact the overdetermination of actions such as these is typical. In this particular case, for example, the re-enactment of the wedding night where the new husband tried again and again to penetrate his bride likely also contributed to the repetition of the symptomatic act.

Let's now look at this patient's second conative attitude. Note that the very same seemingly senseless repetitive symptomatic phantasy action with the maid and the red-stained tablecloth fits also with the second wish or desire—to leave her husband, but only if doing so would not reveal his impotence.[17] Because Freud's text does not indicate the sequence of this symptomatic action in the course of her marriage—whether it preceded her temporarily leaving him or whether it occurred after she decided to stay—two different interpretations are plausible. If the symptom was first, the showing of the "red stain" actually meant she could leave without embarrassing him about his potency, and so she really left. Thus, both the symptomatic action and the action that followed suggest desire rather than wish, if the symptom occurred first. But what if the symptom post-dated her decision to stay? The presence of the symptom suggests that she was still ambivalent about what was now even more unacceptable regarding leaving him. Unacceptable, but she could still *do* it: "see there's the 'red stain'; his potency is fine." We should conclude here too, that desire is the likely conative attitude because it seems she cannot, as a less neurotic (but perhaps equally unhappy) person might, reconcile her decision to stay with a continued wish (mere wish, perhaps with wish-fulfilling phantasy, but requiring no action) to go. Instead the unhappy wife stays, simultaneously and repetitively performing the symptomatic action that would meet the condition allowing her to fulfill her desire to leave.

Finally, there is the desire of which the patient is aware—the bizarre desire to show the stain to the housemaid. This desire is a condensed substitute and a disguise both for the impossible first desire—that on their wedding night he had deflowered her successfully with blood stains to prove it; and the ambivalently held and unacceptable second desire—that she can leave him and do so without impugning his masculinity because the maid can attest to his potency. This third desire can be fulfilled, and it is, repetitively. But, to the extent it is only a cover-up, actions satisfying this desire will of course do no work toward fulfilling the two desires underlying it.[18]

The account of the constitutive function of desire offered in this chapter, along with a recognition of the confounding of conative attitudes wish and desire, have helped clarify two interesting psychoanalytic/philosophy of action

---

[17] The economy of mental operations is organized so that one such symptomatic action often pertains to many conflicts. This obviates what would be a great deal of mental work in designing a multitude of symptoms. (See Freud, SE, Vols 4 and 5, 1900; SE, Vol. 20, 1926.)

[18] In fact continually fulfilling the third desire interferes with this patient becoming aware of what would be a more normal desire to understand her troubled marriage.

cases. In addition two long-standing psychoanalytic questions have been addressed; possibly even answered. First, why do external actions follow from what seem to be internally gratifiable wishes? Second, why do so many neurotic actions occur repetitively? The next case is as puzzling from the standpoint of psychoanalytic theory as it is commonplace in psychoanalytic practice.

Case 3: Wish as a defense against desire

Why do patients who have wishes they deem unacceptable—wishes they know they will never act upon—nonetheless experience conscious guilt over these wishes and/or neurotic symptoms that seem to have these wishes as their cause? A typical case follows: A professional man in his mid-twenties, Mr J has a highly conflictual relationship with his mother. He knows that he hates her some of the time. At these times he consciously knows that he wishes she were dead, moreover that he wishes to kill her. Even at these times however, he also knows that he would not act in any way to hasten his mother's death. Not only is he aware that he sometimes loves her, but any homicidal act (including any act of omission that would not befit a decent son) would tear him from his life as he knows it. Still, Mr J suffers from conscious guilt and a variety of self-punishing symptoms, all of which clearly seem to result from these murderous wishes toward his mother. The most striking symptom is a self-disabling he effects whenever he engages in any activity he construes to be aggressively competitive with an older woman. His boss is an older woman, and this symptom has occurred repetitively in her presence such that he has compromised his success at work. When both he and his boss are together at a meeting and both have opinions to offer, he will do one of three things: he will forget the meeting, come unprepared, or become inarticulate almost to the point of incoherence as he tries to express his ideas. Although usually a good worker, with a better than average capacity for self-expression, Mr J repeatedly manages to be incompetent whenever others evaluate him and his boss head to head.

So what is going on here? He "knows" he has an unacceptable wish that he also "knows" is "just a wish" and yet he has guilt and crippling symptoms. Solving the puzzle begins by noticing the repetitive nature of his symptomatic actions. Is it the case here as in the prior example, that instead of a wish, some insistent and persistent desire—with its constitutive function ever-producing a readiness-to-act toward fulfilling the desire's content—is the likely conative attitude motivating these symptomatic acts? If so, what desire? The simplest answer is the correct one, namely, that Mr J desires to kill his mother. This is obviously an unacceptable desire and would lead to unacceptable actions and consequences. And so it is not so surprising that Mr J remains totally unaware of this desire-as-a-desire, even as he is fully conscious of the content in the wish form. In other words Mr J, not through any conscious mechanism, disguises his unrelenting and terrible desire by experiencing it and treating it as a totally harmless wish.

But even though the murderous desire is unconscious and disguised as a conscious wish, since desires press for actions, various real-world actions, including some behavioral manifestations of internal changes, do take place. Whereas matricide is short-circuited, (1) Mr J pleads guilty to a lesser charge (disabling or manslaughter rather than murder). (2) He also changes the victim of this crime from his mother to himself, as he acts to disable himself. (3) He makes matricide impossible anyway as he is so incompetent. And, finally (4) Mr J punishes himself for his matricidal desires nevertheless, with his self-defeating actions at work and with his guilt. The symptoms and the guilt experienced by this patient become understandable once we consider that he suffers from an unacceptable but relentless (unconscious) desire, not a mere wish.

Case 4: Revisiting the Rat Man

Many of the problems from which Freud's (1909, pp. 151–318) famous patient, the Rat Man, suffered were ascribed to dangerously powerful wishes—wishes Freud termed omnipotent. The *omnipotence of wishes (and thoughts)* explored in depth in the Rat Man case, became quite important in Freud's general theorizing. An omnipotent wish can be simply characterized. An agent holds that merely wishing X will result in X happening, without any real-world activity on the agent's part. Described by Freud as a species of the more general phenomenon of *overvaluation of thought*, such thinking alone is believed by agents engaged in this overvaluation to be sufficient to cause material changes. A philosophical conative attitude analysis can add another dimension to understanding this psychoanalytic concept.

The Rat Man, out of ambivalence toward his beloved, moved a stone out of the way of her carriage so that the carriage would come to no harm. Later, recognizing that his action was absurd, he moved the stone back to its original spot (1909, p. 191). Freud maintains that the Rat Man was acting to protect his lady from his wishful but ambivalently held unconscious "hostile impulses." This seems right; I want only to put a finer point on Freud's analysis by proposing that these impulses were part of an unconscious *desire* the Rat Man had that she would come to harm, not a wish. In my view, it is because desire leads to action that his hostility necessitated the counteraction of moving the stone out of the carriage's path. Next he performed another action counter to the counteraction—moving the stone back to its original location—demonstrating with this second action both his original hostility and his recognition of the irrationality of his first act. It is interesting to note that although the Rat Man, like Mr J above in Case 3, was fully aware of the violent content—the Rat Man was obsessed with his lady coming to harm—he was totally unaware that he *desired* to harm her. In fact the Rat Man was unaware that he had any conative attitude with that content, much less that he had a readiness-to-act aimed at harming her.

I state above that he had an unconscious desire to harm her and not a wish. I want to emend this. He had a desire to harm her; not a wish—at least not an *ordinary wish*. Perhaps the Rat Man's conative attitude could be best described in Freud's terms as an omnipotent wish or omnipotent thought. On Freud's account patients hold that their omnipotent wishes or thoughts cause actions (with deleterious consequences) without any real-world action by the patient. In other words the Rat Man's very thought that his lady's carriage would topple over could magically cause just such an accident. Given this view, patients like the Rat Man need to defend against any actions that might become associated with their omnipotent thoughts/wishes too. And so on this basis too, the Rat Man's actions with the stone might be explained.

But concluding that we are unable to determine whether the troubling conative attitude in question for the Rat Man was a persistent (unconscious and unacceptable) desire or an omnipotent wish/thought does not constitute a satisfactory philosophical conative attitude analysis. In an attempt to resolve this problem, I propose that the two phenomena in question are really two different aspects of the same phenomenon. The omnipotent wish captures and describes that which an agent subjectively experiences. For example, patients can feel they have done nothing at all—just wished, maybe even just thought—and yet the content can magically come to pass. Experiencing a conative attitude thus, as an omnipotent wish/thought, a patient can "rightly" deny his/her own activity toward its fulfillment. The unrelenting persistence of unconscious, unacceptable desire, on the other hand, while not experienced by the agent at all, provides an underlying mechanism and explanation for repetitive actions that would otherwise seem bizarrely incoherent.[19] The Rat Man not

---

[19] The Rat Man's symptomatic actions provide a very clear demonstration of Freud's three assumptions at work—psychic continuity, psychic determinism, and a meaningful, dynamic unconscious. Moving the stone twice looks incoherent. Assuming psychic continuity and determinism, we know there will be a psychologically meaningful cause. Conscious reasons and explanations fall short. But in positing an unconscious hostile desire—and the ever-readiness-to-act toward its fulfillment, which is a desire's constitutive

only omnipotently thought about harm to his lady, he desired (unconsciously) to hurt her, and he desired (consciously) to keep her safe. Thus, he moved the stone out of the way, and then performed the counteraction of moving it back into the way. Action and counteraction taken together were both in accord with defending against his "omnipotent" fully conscious hostile thought *and* his unacceptable unconscious desire.[20]

Case 5: The problem of akrasia

Akrasia, or weakness of the will, has been discussed by philosophers at least as far back as Aristotle. Donald Davidson (1970a, pp. 21–42) gives the modern standard version of the dilemma of the akratic person. A man has a desire for *a* and is able to do *a*. He also has a desire for *b* and could do *b*. He is free to do *a* or do *b*, and they are mutually exclusive. After taking everything possible into account, he judges that *b* is the better action. On this basis he desires to do *b* more and therefore decides to do *b*. Yet he performs *a* and does not perform *b*. Davidson (p. 42) asks, "what is the agent's reason for doing *a* when he believes it would be better, all things considered, to do another thing [?]." He (p. 42) continues "the answer must be: for this the agent has no reason." In other words although "[o]f course he has a reason for doing *a*; what he lacks is a reason for not letting his better reason for not doing *a* prevail" (p. 42, n. 25). To the extent that the akrate performs akratic actions, he is for Davidson not rational. Further, according to Davidson, the akrate "cannot understand himself: he recognizes in his own internal behavior, something essentially surd" (p. 42).

Let us investigate this with an example that is both specific and commonplace. H drinks sugary soft drinks, and colas are his favorite. He knows, all things considered, that it is better not to drink them. Thus with each can or bottle of cola, he both desires to drink it—let us say he desires *a*; and desires not to drink it—let us call this his desire for *b*. Not drinking colas would be better, and *b* is

---

function to produce—the need for repetitive defensive action and the incoherent-seeming behavior is rendered quite understandable.

[20] One final remark on the Rat Man: As stated above, the Rat Man was not aware of *any* pro-attitude regarding the content, "harm to his lady." (In this way he was unlike Mr J of Case 3.) The Rat Man did not *consciously* desire, wish, or hope that this state of affairs be brought about in the world. He merely thought obsessively about harm coming her way, and indeed consciously *feared* that this state of affairs would be brought about. Fear, in this context, is a mental attitude psychoanalysts routinely understand as a fear of one's own (unconscious, omnipotently powerful hostile) wishes. This fits for the Rat Man, but we should add that he feared no less his (unconscious) hostile *desire* with its readiness-to-act toward fulfillment in the real world of its violent content.

the better act. Therefore, according to Davidson, H should desire *b* more. Yet H continues to imbibe cola soft drinks—he does *a*, he does not do *b*.

Davidson's problem can be addressed fairly readily if one considers readiness-to-act as desire's constitutive function and the psychological calculus alluded to earlier in this chapter. An agent's *judgment* that an action *b* is better than some other action *a*, even all things considered, is no assurance, Davidson's (1970a, p. 23) claim to the contrary not withstanding, that this agent will *desire* *b* more than *a*. This type of example makes it clear that desire and evaluative judgment are not intrinsically linked. To desire something does not mean, as Davidson claims, that one has an attitude toward it as worthy of that desire.[21] Rather, on my view, desire's constitutive function of readiness-to-act links it to intentional action such that if an agent performs desired action *a* intentionally and does not perform desired action *b*, no matter what other factors are considered, in some sense he can be said to desire *a* more. H judges that *b*, stopping cola drinking, is better. But H does *a*, he drinks colas. Hence, H desires *a* more. Note that this analysis does not preclude H having a strong wish for *b*, to stop imbibing colas, even as he does *a*, and drinks them. Moreover, H might well have a strong wish that he could desire *b* more than he desires *a*. In fact, just these sorts of conflict between wish and desire is likely present in every case of akrasia.[22] And yet, as long as he continues to do *a*, his cola drinking is reflective of his stronger desire and its constitutive aim of readiness-to-act in the real world toward fulfillment of its content.

---

[21] People do however try to arrange things such that it seems (especially to themselves) that their evaluative judgments come out right. For example a cola drinker says, "I know it is better all things considered to quit. But it is better *now* to drink this one cola, because it will help sharpen my focus in this important situation. And I can stop drinking colas tomorrow."

[22] The example, at the beginning of this chapter, of one sibling's hope for another's good performance on a Latin exam can be revisited in light of these views on akrasia. Take the case of Sibling A, who hopes Sibling B does well, but does nothing in terms of helping him. Suppose now that A had judged that it would have been better to help B. We can still say that Sibling A's hope functioned as a mere wish; but we might wonder if Sibling A also had a *desire* (conscious or unconscious) that Sibling B *not do well*. If so, this desire would have lead to the action of inhibiting active helping. Some akratic cases may be similar. The smoker judges it would be better to stop smoking and he hopes to stop; but this hope is functioning at the level of mere wish, perhaps because there is also an unconscious *desire* of a self-destructive nature, in addition to the desire to smoke, which together add up to continued smoking. (I owe the idea that Sibling A might have a desire that Sibling B not do well to Howard Shevrin, personal communication.)

Cases 4 and 5 are instructive; they suggest that accompanying every omnipotent wish (and thought) and many akratic acts are *unconscious* desires, often forbidden or unacceptable. In these two cases as in all five, it becomes clear that understanding the role of unconscious desire, constitutively functioning to aid in the production of readiness-to-act toward fulfillment of its own content, is central to an increased understanding of various problem cases in psychoanalysis and the philosophy of action. Further, all five cases suggest that belief/desire analyses as usually done are inadequate and must include not only other propositional attitudes such as wish and phantasy, but also propositional attitudes both conscious and unconscious. Finally, the account of desire's constitutive function proposed in this chapter explains some vexing aspects of clinical psychoanalytic theory including: (1) the repetitive nature of symptomatic acts, (2) the need for symptomatic external actions when it seems that internally gratifying phantasies should suffice, (3) why "harmless" wishes occasion symptoms, and (4) the complex relation between omnipotent wishes (and thoughts) and unconscious desires.

Conclusions (mostly directed to psychoanalysts)

My discussion of wishes not linked to action-readiness may seem jarring (or just plain wrong) to psychoanalysts. Freud did not distinguish the terms "desire" from "wish," and used "wish" much more extensively. As such for him wishes were intimately related to drives and their active striving for discharge. What I have proposed does not so much disagree with this aspect of Freud's view, as extend it developmentally. I have held that earlier in development there is no difference between wish and desire, and that the operative conative attitude is some combination. But that later, as a person matures, this undifferentiated conative attitude is made distinct such that desires are linked to action-readiness, while wishes are experienced and treated differently—they are "mere" wishes, seeking their fulfillment in harmless phantasy. This distinction takes a good deal of maturation just as is true for distinguishing between the cognitive attitudes of phantasy and belief. It is my view that in proposing this distinction, which fits the developmental facts, psychoanalytic concepts are sharpened in a fashion that meaningfully allows a better understanding of some heretofore puzzling psychoanalytic and philosophical cases.

Part V

Summary and conclusions

This part will consist of two chapters. Chapter 9, "Compare and contrast: Gardner, Lear, Cavell, and Brakel," will provide a contrastive summary of the views presented here with three important works in the interdisciplinary area of psychoanalytic theory and the philosophy of mind and action. In so doing Chapter 9 will indicate the major themes of the current volume, leading to Chapter 10, "Summary and conclusions."

Chapter 9

Compare and contrast

Gardner, Lear, Cavell, and Brakel[1]

As I mentioned in Chapter 1, "Introduction," there are many books on philosophy and psychoanalysis. In this chapter I will take up three important such
volumes (1) to illustrate the differences between each of these books and the
present work, highlighting the advantages my contribution affords; and (2) to
begin to provide an overview summary of the account I have proposed.

Sebastian Gardner

Sebastian Gardner's 1993 book *Irrationality and the Philosophy of Psychoanalysis*,
for the purpose of contrasting it with the current volume, can be understood as
advancing four major points, the first two of which I am in total agreement.
They are:

(1) Irrationality (the phenomena and the behavior) can be best explained by
    psychoanalysis and psychoanalytic theory (p. 1). Implied here for both
    Gardner and me, is that irrational acts, events, thoughts, symptoms must
    be taken seriously, and be given a full and adequate account. Too often in
    academic psychology and in philosophy, irrationality is taken to reflect
    mistakes in rationality, something to be accounted for simply and on a case
    by case basis.

(2) Psychoanalysis need not be a psychology of part-minds, or a psychology of
    second minds or second persons in order to account for unconscious men-
    tation. Here (pp. 40–84) Gardner takes issue with Sartre's second mind
    theory, where the second mind is a censor. He also argues against the
    second mind and part-person conceptions of both Pears and Davidson.[2]

---

[1] I thank three anonymous reviewers for suggesting the inclusion of the material in this
chapter.

[2] I have briefly addressed Davidson's view on this in Chapter 5.

On Gardner's next two points and what follows from them, he and I sharply disagree. Gardner (1993) argues that:

(3) Psychoanalysis is not, what he terms, Ordinary Psychology, but is an *extension* of Ordinary Psychology (e.g. pp. 5–6, 7–10, 116–18, 123, 188). For Gardner Ordinary Psychology can explain ordinary conflicts— i.e. conflicts between desires, among the contents of desires, and among aspects of desires and beliefs—and it can even explain the mildly irrational self-deceptions and akrasias. However, Gardner maintains that Ordinary Psychology cannot explain deeply irrational neurotic symptoms. This is because for Gardner neurotic symptoms are not conflicts between propositional attitudes or among their contents (pp. 90–5). Rather, neurotic symptoms consist in troublesome pre-propositional components (p. 104, 110) and they are thereby heterogeneous with respect to ordinary conflicts.

While this understanding of neurotic symptoms helps Gardner (pp. 101–4) develop a cogent notion of repression—the mechanism both keeps pre-propositional components unconscious, and causes unacceptable, disruptive, and/or difficult propositional mental states to "disintegrate into more primitive, *pre-propositional components*" (p. 104)—it leads him in a more problematic direction, which I will address forthwith.

(4) Since Gardner's view of neurosis already necessitates an extension of Ordinary Psychology and the introduction of additional ontologic entities— for example, the pre-propositional components comprising neurotic symptoms—he must turn to the Kleinian school of psychoanalysis to find a version of psychoanalytic theory that, owing to its own idiosyncrasies, will not just accommodate, but will actually embrace the expanded ontology. (In addition to unconscious pre-propositional phantasies, the added psychological entities include unconscious pre-propositional wishes, and objectless drives [p. 117, 123]). But there is a cost. Since these pre-propositional Kleinian phantasies, and so on are not agential, intentional, or motivational, Gardner must go to great lengths (see pp. 191–3) to explain what can be accounted for rather simply when phantasies, viewed as propositional attitudes, conscious or unconscious, are considered fully agential sources of unconscious intentionality and motivation. (See Chapters 5–8 of this volume.)

On my view, in acknowledging unconscious, irrational, and a-rational mentation, there is no need for the extra metaphysical entities Gardner offers— no need to posit special pre-propositional mental states, and no need for wishes, drives, phantasies that are somehow non-intentional, non-agential. Instead, throughout this book I have made much of primary process a-rational thought, both in its formal operations and in its contents, comprising various types of propositional attitudes, conscious and unconscious, including those of which neurotic symptoms and irrational behavior consist.

While I strongly agree with Gardner that irrationality must be accounted for, and that this can be best done by psychoanalytic theory, I strongly disagree with holding psychoanalysis as a special psychology thereby removing it from the realm of ordinary scientific theories. Psychoanalytic data, including those very evident in neuroses and other forms of irrationality, are part of the regular world; and psychoanalytic theory is the specialized, but regular psychological/scientific theory best able to address these intriguing data.[3]

Jonathan Lear

I intend here to discuss only selected aspects of but one of the works of Jonathan Lear, his 1998 book, *Open Minded*. In this work the primary processes and irrationality are centrally featured. The primary processes are for Lear, as for me, active, intrinsic aspects of our mental life; truly "primary" and basic, quite different from the secondary processes. (Marcia Cavell, whom I will discuss next, has a different view.) Further, both Lear and I agree that not only is it the case that secondary process reasoning *is* used defensively to try to rationalize irrational acts and phantasies, but that secondary process rationality *must* be used to reinterpret primary process contents. This owes to a striking quality of human nature: we are self-interpreting animals who need, as much as want to seem rational to others and especially to ourselves. (See e.g. Lear 1998, pp. 101, 109, 113–14; and the current work, Chapters 4, 7, and 8.)

But Lear and I part company as to the nature of primary process phantasies. Since they are nonrational, Lear seems not even to consider the possibility that they could be propositional attitudes. This view aligns Lear with Gardner and the Kleinian school, and saddles his account with all the problems attendant thereof, discussed just above.

Then there is another problem with Lear's account, and it concerns a confounding of the a-rational with the irrational.[4] On my view primary process a-rational thinking is not synonymous with irrational thinking, nor does it necessarily lead to irrational behavior. Elsewhere (Brakel and Shevrin 2003)

---

[3] Insofar as mine is the simpler view, entailing no special entities and no special science to explain them, my account offers an advantage over Gardner's.

[4] Actually this is not just Lear's problem; many, maybe most theorists, confound the a-rational with the irrational.

I have proposed that primary process, a-rational thinking might in fact be the predominant mode in higher mammals and birds, and that far from being irrational, in the sense of rationality gone wrong, a-rational mentation could represent an evolutionarily successful means of thinking. (See also the current work, Chapter 5.)

But psychoanalytic theorists such as Lear might say, how can this a-rational/irrational distinction work for psychoanalytically relevant problems—if some behavior or propositional attitude is a-rational, isn't it necessarily irrational for human agents? The answer is no, and in the current work I have proposed the following explanation. Irrationality, say in the form of neurotic symptoms, results, in simplest form, from agents unconsciously disguising and yet expressing unacceptable phantasies, wishes or desires (which themselves can be rational, a-rational, or irrational) using primary process a-rational means and mechanisms such as displacement, condensation, part-for-whole, and so on. The primary processes and their a-rational means are in this way appropriated to an end result that often consists in frankly irrational behavior, made even more irrational by the agent's need to construe the behavior as justifiable and rational. But at other times and in other situations these very same a-rational primary process operations (displacement, condensation, and part-for-whole) can be used toward reasonable ends, for example, in creative endeavors of all sorts, and in deriving novel solutions to problems in many domains.

Thus Lear's position, like Gardner's, adds unnecessary entities to the ontology of the mental. Meanwhile his view, by constraining the primary processes to the realm of the irrational, provides a less than satisfying account of this a-rational form of mentation, its contents and various functional roles.

Marcia Cavell

In *The Psychoanalytic Mind: From Freud to Philosophy*, Marcia Cavell (1993) presents a position on irrationality and primary process that owes much to the work of Donald Davidson. Like Davidson, Cavell is a meaning holist for whom rationality is constitutive of the mental (p. 201). I will not rehearse the arguments made in Chapter 5 against this view, but instead will outline briefly what these commitments entail for Cavell.

(1) Primary process is parasitic upon secondary process and not merely epistemologically[5] (pp. 174–5). Indeed for Cavell primary process mentation

---

5 Discovering primary process, knowing it, does require secondary process. This epistemic dependence is uncontested and unproblematic. Freud, for example, repeatedly observed that something quite different from ordinary rationality was operative in many of the

can be only: (i) proto-secondary process—as for example in the young, who have not yet developed their secondary process capacities sufficiently, or (ii) pathologically regressed versions of secondary process thinking— that is, in adults, thinkers fully capable of secondary process thinking, the primary processes serve a largely defensive function, fending off content troubling to these mostly rational agents. In both cases primary process is ontologically and even conceptually dependent upon secondary process mentation. This constitutive dependence is very different from the accounts given by Gardner and Lear, as well as the one in the present work.

(2) Not surprisingly, on Cavell's view phantasy too, as it is rich in primary process content, has a much more limited role. It is largely defensive, taking agents away from anxiety (pp. 187–91).

(3) Irrationality does arise when primary process operations and phantasies work on anxiety-laden thoughts from childhood. But just as is true in the Davidsonian picture, for Cavell the irrational aspects are partitioned off from, and inaccessible to the holistic network of rational secondary process thoughts (pp. 202–03). Cavell's position, of course, inherits all of the problems of divided mind accounts of unconsciousness and irrational-ity. (As discussed above, Gardner takes these problems up at length, and I do briefly in Chapter 5.)

(4) Children are proto-rational with proto-secondary process concepts and categories instead of primary process concepts and categories (pp. 168–9, 203–4).

Cavell's problematic views stem from her Davidsonian position that rationality is constitutive of the mental. Thus, irrationality on Cavell's account can occupy but a small role, and *a-rationality* does not seem to even get a bit part. While the notion that rational normativity constitutes the mental can be of instru-mental help in providing a justification for psychoanalytic interpretation— the analyst assumes that the patient can be rational, helping the patient to see the gaps and deviations in his/her associations—it does exactly *no work* in properly understanding the ontology of the mental. Holding rationality as

thought processes of young children, in the formation of dreams and psychological symp-toms, and in his patients' free associations. From here he appreciated the systematic nature of these differences, and "posited" the primary processes. Psychoanalysts routinely go through the same stages when hearing free associative material at odds with secondary process rationality. Indeed this epistemic priority may help in guiding and justifying specific psychoanalytic interpretations made at given times to particular patients.

constitutive of the mental instead begs a vital question; it assumes that the ontology of the mental is identical with its epistemology.

Having provided a brief look at some major contrasts and comparisons between the views presented in this book and those of Sebastian Gardner, Jonathan Lear, and Marcia Cavell, including some advantages my position affords, I will now proceed to the final chapter for a more general summary and some conclusions.

Chapter 10

Summary and conclusions

Goals of an interdisciplinary approach

In each of the chapters of this book I have taken an area directly related to one or more of the central tenets of psychoanalysis and provided a philosophical analysis. One of the goals in this endeavor was to demonstrate the advantages of using this interdisciplinary approach to both psychoanalysis and to the philosophies of mind and action. Let us look first at the gains for psychoanalysis.

Psychoanalytic general theory is a beautiful and elegant theory—one with a total theory of mind derivable from very few basic posits: the assumptions of psychic continuity, psychic determinism, and a meaningful dynamic psychological unconscious, the application of the technique of free association, and the corollary of mentation organized according to both primary and secondary process principles. But psychoanalytic theory is neither very well understood, nor very popular, in these early years of the twenty-first century. Partly owing to competitive pressure in all areas of mental health to demonstrate improved clinical applications and rapid treatment outcomes, emphasis, interest, and above all critical attention to the theory has fallen off sharply. Hence, the increased conceptual concision offered in these chapters, focused on basic concepts tied closely to the most fundamental principles of psychoanalysis, clearly represents an effort to reverse this trend. If this endeavor is successful, it could be of great benefit to psychoanalytic general theory, both practically, through leading to better reception in the academic world outside of psychoanalytic institutes, and even more importantly, intrinsically, improving it as a general theory of mind. Along the latter lines of thought, as has been shown in many of these chapters, psychoanalytic theory can gain convergent support from its neighboring disciplines—the philosophies of mind and action; and as is true for any theory, psychoanalytic general theory can only be strengthened by the demonstration of such convergences.

With respect to philosophy, the main advantage of the interdisciplinary approach used in this book concerns extending the domain of interest. Beyond the relatively narrow confines of conscious and rational mentation, and conscious and rationally mediated intentional action, the interdisciplinary approach favored in this book, offers the opportunity for a philosophy of mind and a philosophy of action that can deal also with unconscious, a-rational, and irrational mentation, and intentional action so mediated. The standard way of dealing with a-rational or irrational behaviors is to consider such behaviors mistakes, rare glitches in our usual rational functioning.[1] But to regard such a large sweep of human goings-on in this restricted, circumscribed, almost parenthetical matter cannot serve philosophy well. For, after all, our desires to the contrary notwithstanding, so much of what we think, who we are, and what we do cannot be adequately described, much less understood, in terms of consciousness and rationality alone.

Rationality: Iterations of the human tendency

But what I claim to be a limiting focus in mainstream philosophy of mind and action reflects, in a formalized and scholarly fashion, an aspect of a universal human tendency: We want to see ourselves (and our fellow humans) as ever conscious, rational, and "in the know." This tendency is iterative, it occurs on many levels, and is a major theme throughout this book. The title of Chapter 2, for example, asks a question, "What sort of a theory is psychoanalytic theory?" The answer is that it is an unusual theory because it is a theory about unconscious and primary process mentation—mentation we cannot know consciously and mentation that does not meet criteria for rationality. Thus, given the human tendency to characterize everything in rational terms, it is not surprising that the first task in Chapter 2 is to address two different skeptical views on which the very concepts of unconscious and primary process representations are characterized as either incoherent or otiose. These skeptics "argue"—really they present "by definition" assertions more than argument—that only what is rational and conscious can be considered psychological, therefore what is a-rational and/or unconscious cannot. I have tried to defeat the skeptics conservatively, using failings in their own arguments. However, it is also the case that accepting the sort of reductive ontology of the mental that these skeptics recommend would occasion giving up on explaining

---

[1] See Stanovich and West 2001, for a thoroughgoing presentation on recent philosophical and research psychology accounts of dual processes of thinking. Prominent in this work is the prevailing view that a-rational and irrational thinking and behavior are due to cognitive processing errors and/or other sorts of mistakes. But see Brakel and Shevrin 2003, for a commentary on this article. We take issue with the mainstream views and offer an alternative account in line with the views presented in this book.

in psychological terms so many human transactions, interactions, strivings, conflicts, and behaviors—so much of what is human.

Chapter 3 shows Kant to have regarded associationism as an organizing mental principle far before Freud's similar claim that primary process principles, including association, are the first organizers of our mental life. And yet Kant claimed that what was necessary for any human understanding and even any human experience was that his secondary process type "categories" mediate our mental organization. Again the rational predominates.

In Chapter 4, we can see the very same human tendency toward inexorable secondary process rationalizing in the report of dreams. Dreams while dreamt, for the majority of dreamers most of the time, provide a highly convincing demonstration of material organized in a primary process fashion. And yet the dreams-as-dreamt routinely undergo a secondary process revision and/or re-elaboration as they become the dream material we remember and recount after awakening. The secondary process re-configuring, whatever other functions (e.g. defensive disguise) it may or may not have, provides a structure for us *to be able to* remember and recount them.

Chapter 4 also addresses another aspect of our human desire to "be in the know," helping to explain why primary process mentation is hard to know. Not only is primary process material automatically (and unconsciously) recast into secondary process form in order for secondary process thinkers to *know of it* as well as to *know it at all*, but persons in primary process mental states— where contents are not regulated with respect to truth conditions obtaining in the world—are not actually capable of meeting criteria for believing, much less knowing. This is a very unstable situation for human cognizers, and were we to know and properly categorize ourselves as being in such primary process mental states, we would be most uncomfortable.

In Chapter 5, we again see doubts raised about the coherence of the concept of primary process contents, as the work of the attributionist philosophers take the universal human desire to regard ourselves (and others) as knowledgeable and rational to new heights. Demonstrating the human proclivity to see rationality (almost) everywhere, this group of philosophers attributes holistic rationality charitably to (almost) everyone (almost) all of the time. They then claim that content can only be constituted by successful (rational) interpretation of such rational actors (or speakers). This has two consequences. One is very expectable—meaningful content is understood as meaningful only if rational interpreters can know it. The other consequence is most radical—the very constitution of meaningful content as content is dependent on rational interpreters knowing it. Thus assuming I am properly rational and a good enough interpreter, *if I cannot know some content as content, it does not exist as content.*

The ontological takes a back seat to the epistemological, as *rational interpretive success is constitutive of mental content*. Of course, under these constraints, primary process and unconscious contents are gone—in fact they never did exist, except as incoherent concepts!

Chapters 7 and 8 deal with clinical topics, clearly quite different from the matters taken up in Chapter 5. And yet the material in these final clinical chapters continues to show the human tendency to regard that which is rational and can be consciously known as coextensive with what exists. In these chapters we see patients mistyping their propositional attitudes toward the rational and the conscious. In Chapter 7, patients can be better understood, once we realize that they are experiencing and treating their "neurotic-beliefs"—highly irrational phantasies with unconscious and conflictual components kept in place with spurious psychic-reality testing—as though they were rational beliefs-proper, cognitive attitudes highly constrained by constitutively aiming at the truth. And in Chapter 8, we see that patients must convince themselves that they have conscious unacceptable "wishes"—mere wishes that they would never act upon—rather than dangerous unconscious desires. Desires, because of their link to action, are far more dangerous than wishes, especially unconscious desires where people do not feel in rational control of their own actions.

Primary process content

Since the programmatic aim of this book is utilizing an interdisciplinary approach toward mutual advantage for psychoanalytic theory and the philosophies of mind and action, the central piece of this work concerns making a philosophical case for primary process content. Part III, Chapter 5 is entirely devoted to this task, a task essential not just for my project, but for Freud's general theory of mind—particularly Corollary One, which regards the primary processes, not just the secondary processes, as truly mental and contentful. As primary process mentation is not rational but a-rational, the argument for primary process mentation necessitates something other than rational normativity and interpretative success in order to fix content. As primary process mentation does not occur in the form of conscious beliefs/conscious desire, something different from the standard belief/desire propositional attitude analysis is also needed. Thus, I advanced a proper function account for the primary processes in the propositional attitude form phantasy/wish in which they occur, such that selective fitness success and evolutionary normativity (rather than interpretative success and rational normativity) can constitute the determinate content of particular primary process mental states.

The implications of successfully fixing content for the primary processes in this way are important. First, proper function accounts can be applied to other aspects of psychoanalytic theory, as was demonstrated in Chapter 6 on drive objects. And perhaps of even greater moment, given the success of the argument in Chapter 5, psychoanalytic theory can claim a philosophical grounding for the concept of contentful primary process mentation.

The inadequacy of belief/desire accounts of human psychology

That the argument for primary process content necessitated propositional attitudes outside the usual conscious belief/desire analysis proves important generally. In several chapters in this book, it was demonstrated that to account adequately for human motivation, intention, and behavior, considerations limited to an agent's conscious beliefs and conscious desires cannot suffice. Other propositional attitudes were therefore introduced into the analyses and explanations of motivated human behavior—phantasy and wish in Chapter 5, instinctual drive in Chapter 6, and neurotic-belief, essentially a complicated unconscious phantasy, in Chapter 7. In Chapter 8, the importance of including *unconscious* desire became manifest—cases considered puzzling remained so until the role of unconscious desire was uncovered.

Determinate, albeit not singular

The proper function account for primary process content in the form of phantasies and wishes given in Chapter 5 also provided a useful template for a related proper function account for the objects of drives. Drive objects are such that they cannot be represented singularly, yet it is obvious they cannot be considered indeterminate. The key to resolving this apparent problem comes in recognizing that the satisfiers of each drive, although not singular, can instead be seen as constituting a single set or category whose members share some primary process attribute or feature. With drive objects seen as such primary process organized categories—rather than as random assortments—a proper function account of drive objects follows naturally. Important in itself for the understanding of the nature of drive objects, this proper function account also allows a distinction to be made between what is indeterminate without content, and what is not singular but nonetheless determinate and contentful. This distinction bears on the philosophical issue of vagueness. I conclude Chapter 6 arguing that the resemblance between vague concepts and primary process-linked concepts is strictly superficial, finding once again that the impetus to equate them was predicated on the all-too-human tendency to regard as inadequate any concept that is not organized according to rational secondary process categories.

Clinical theory puzzles

In addition to the overarching aim of an interdisciplinary approach with mutual advantage to the philosophies of mind and action and general psycho-analytic theory, I count among the goals of this book an attempt to justify taking as true the fundamental posits of psychoanalytic theory. Why would one want to do that? Only because when the foundational posits of the psycho-analytic theory of mind are taken as true, puzzling examples of human motiva-tions, intentions, and behaviors can be better understood. Conversely, when these fundamentals of psychoanalytic theory are not taken as true, much remains seemingly unexplainable. But obviously, neither of these facts, nor both together, can provide grounds for the justification sought. Thus, Chapter 2 advances an argument for taking-as-true the foundations of psychoanalytic theory based on analogy with arguments concerning the geometry of space; and Chapters 3 and 4 provide convergent evidence for the basic assumptions of psychoanalytic theory in Kantian epistemology. These are important and necessary steps.[2]

However and in addition, the clinical chapters of this book revealed an extra and unpredicted sort of justification for taking the foundational posits of psychoanalysis as true—one more internal to psychoanalytic theory. Namely, the fact that certain discoveries about *psychoanalytic clinical theory* follow directly from the philosophical analyses of *psychoanalytic general theory*, implies an underlying internal theoretic cohesion which affords greater confi-dence in the theories at both levels. Thus, for example, while it is not surprising that a philosophical understanding of the nature of unconscious desire would lead to a better understanding of akratic acts, or that a philosophical analysis of primary process drive objects would deepen and even change one's under-standing of the drives and their objects; it is surprising that an analysis of

---

[2] Convergent evidence for (or against) the assumptions of psychoanalytic general theory must also be sought in the domain of empirical scientific investigation. In this sort of research, methods which do not presuppose psychoanalytic presuppositions must be used to test psychoanalytic presuppositions. Our research team (see Chapter 2, footnote 10) has in this manner been able to provide convergent evidence for (1) a dynamic uncon-scious (Assumption Three)—See Shevrin *et al.* (1992, 1996) and Snodgrass *et al.* (1993); and (2) for the existence of primary process thought organization (Corollary One)— See Brakel (2004) for a summary of this second line of research.

unconscious desire would lead to possible answers to several vexing clinical theory questions: (1) Why do symptomatic actions occur at all when gratification through phantasy would seem to obviate the need for any action? (2) Why are symptomatic actions often so repetitive? (3) Is there a relationship between omnipotent wishes and unconscious desires? If so, what is it?

All of these questions can be answered readily, if one accepts the proposal, derived from a philosophical analysis of desire, that readiness-to-act is desire's constitutive function—and it is the constitutive function of conscious desire and unconscious desire no less.[3] Thus, (1) symptomatic actions follow when the causal conative attitude is an action-ready desire (conscious or unconscious), and not an idle wish. (2) Symptomatic actions, unlike wishes potentially gratifiable in phantasy, are often repetitive when they are driving to fulfill in action an unsatisfiable, impossible, or taboo desire. (3) Omnipotent wishes and unconscious desires are two aspects of the same phenomenon. Agents experience what are actually dangerous unconscious desires as forbidden omnipotent wishes. Among other functions, this keeps hidden the most salient ontological fact about unconscious desires—they are conative attitudes always pressing for action toward fulfillment of their contents, deleterious real-world consequences notwithstanding.

Freud's foundational posits, rationality, and the human tendency revisited

Finally, moving back to the general theory and in particular Freud's fundamental posits, one can see in Freud the same desire to bring everything possible into rational, secondary process understanding in order "to be in the know." There is however a difference—in itself a small difference, but one with huge consequences. Whereas most theorists, and the great majority of people who have dreams and symptoms, use the desire to know to *limit* knowledge of the unconscious, and of content organized according to primary rather than secondary process principles, Freud used the desire to know more *inclusively*. Indeed it took Freud's highly sophisticated and acute secondary process mentation to propose and describe primary process and unconscious mentation. But by making the simple, but radical assumptions that human behavior can be studied as lawfully regular, and then that most breaks in this regularity are only seeming-breaks, with the continuity restorable by positing a dynamic

---

[3] The unconscious aspects can be various. One can be unconscious about the content of a desire and/or one can be unconscious about a desire-as-a-desire. In the latter case one is unconscious about the propositional attitude type.

meaningful unconscious, Freud's desire to be in the know expanded profoundly our understanding of humans and our capacity for human understanding. We should not retreat from Freud's general theory of mind—either by dismissing it as not theoretically rigorous enough, or by the opposite—not giving it the theoretical rigor it is due. This book, pointing the way toward revamping both psychoanalytic general theory and standard views in the philosophies of mind and action—by sharpening the grasp of the former and expanding the reach of the latter—is offered in the spirit of not retreating at all; but instead of going forth, going forward.

References

Abad, V and Guilleminault, C (2004). Review of rapid eye movement behavior sleep disorders. *Current Neurology and Neuroscience Reports*, **4**, 157–63.

Anscombe, GEM (1957). *Intention*, Harvard University Press, Cambridge, MA.

Arlow, J (1985). The concept of psychic reality and related problems. *Journal of the American Psychoanalytic Association*, **33**, 521–35.

Arlow, J (1991a). Derivative manifestations of perversions. In G Fogel, ed. *Perversion and near-perversions in clinical practice*, pp. 59–74. Yale University Press, New Haven.

Arlow, J (1991b). The personal myth. In P Hartocollis, ed. *The personal myth in psychoanalytic theory*, pp. 21–35. International Universities Press, Madison, CT.

Arlow, J (1996). The concept of psychic reality—how useful? *International Journal of Psychoanalysis*, **77**, 659–66.

Baillargeon, R (1987). Young infants' reasoning about the physical and spatial characteristics of a hidden object. *Cognitive Development*, **3**, 179–200.

Barrouillet, P and Markovits, H (2002). Is the self-organizing consciousness framework compatible with human deductive reasoning? Commentary on Perruchet and Vinter (2002). The self-organizing consciousness. *Behavioral and Brain Sciences*, **25**, 330–331.

Bornstein, R (2002) Consciousness organizes more than itself: Findings from subliminal mere exposure research. Commentary on Perruchet and Vinter (2002). The self-organizing consciousness. *Behavioral and Brain Sciences*, **25**, 332–3.

Brakel, LAW (1984). The fate of the dream after awakening: stages toward analytic understanding. *Journal of Evolutionary Psychology*, **5**, 97–108.

Brakel, LAW (1989). Negative hallucinations, other irretrievable experiences and two functions of consciousness. *International Journal of Psychoanalysis*, **70**, 461–79.

Brakel, LAW (1991). Psychoanalytic data: two problems contributing to our evidential difficulties. Presentation, *American Psychological Association Meetings, Division 39*, Chicago, Illinois.

Brakel, LAW (1994a). On knowing the unconscious: lessons from the epistemology of geometry and space. *International Journal of Psycho-Analysis*, **75**, 39–49.

Brakel, LAW (1994b). Book review essay of *The rediscovery of the mind* (1992) by John Searle. *The Psychoanalytic Quarterly*, **63**, 787–92.

Brakel, LAW (2001). Phantasies, neurotic-beliefs, and beliefs-proper. *American Journal of Psychoanalysis*, **61**, 363–89.

Brakel, LAW (2002). Phantasy and wish: a proper function account of a-rational primary process mediated mentation. *Australasian Journal of Philosophy*, **80**, 1–16.

Brakel, LAW (2003). "Unusual" human experiences: Kant, Freud and an associationist law. In *Theoria et Historica Scientificarum*: Special issue on Unconscious perception and communication: evolutionary, cognitive and psychoanalytic perspectives, **7**, 109–16.

Brakel, LAW (2004). The psychoanalytic assumption of the primary process: extra-psychoanalytic evidence and findings. *Journal of the American Psychoanalytic Association*, **2**, 1131–61.

Brakel, LAW (2005). Drive theory and primary process: a philosophical account. In P Giampieri-Deutsch, ed. *Psychoanalysis as an empirical interdisciplinary science: collected papers on contemporary psychoanalytic research*, pp. 75–90. Austrian Academy of Science Press, Vienna.

Brakel, LAW (2007). Music and primary process: proposal for a preliminary experiment. *American Imago*, **64**, 37–57.

Brakel, LAW (forthcoming). Knowledge and belief: psychoanalytic evidence in support of a radical epistemic view. *American Imago*.

Brakel, LAW, Kleinsorge, S, Snodgrass, M, and Shevrin, H (2000). The primary process and the unconscious: experimental evidence supporting two psychoanalytic presuppositions. *International Journal of Psychoanalysis*, **81**, 553–69.

Brakel, LAW, Shevrin, H, and Villa, K (2002). The priority of primary process categorization: experimental evidence supporting a psychoanalytic developmental hypothesis. *Journal of the American Psychoanalytic Association*, **50**, 483–505.

Brakel, LAW and Shevrin, H (2003). Freud's dual process theory and the place of the a-rational. Continuing Commentary on Stanovich and West (2001). Individual differences in reasoning: implications for the rationality debate. *Behavioral and Brain Sciences*, **23**, 645–66, in *Behavioral and Brain Sciences*, **26**, 527–8.

Brakel, LAW and Shevrin, H (2005). Anxiety, attributional thinking and primary process. *International Journal of Psychoanalysis*, **86**, 1679–93.

Bratman, M (1999). *Intention, plans, and practical reason*, CSLI Publications, Stanford.

Brenner, C (1982). *The mind in conflict*, International Universities Press, New York.

Cameron, O and Wimer, LA (1979). An anticholinergic toxicity reaction to chlorpromazine activated by psychological stress. *The Journal of Nervous and Mental Diseases*, **167**, 508–10.

Cavell, M (1993). *The psychoanalytic mind: from freud to philosophy*, Harvard University Press, Cambridge, MA.

Church, J (1987). Reasonable irrationality. *Mind*, **96**, 354–66.

Cherniak, R (1981). Minimal rationality. *Mind*, **90**, 161–83.

Davidson, D (1963). Actions, reasons, and causes. In *Actions and events*, pp. 3–19. Clarendon Press, 1980, Oxford.

Davidson, D (1967) Truth and meaning. In *Truth and interpretation*, pp. 17–36. Clarendon Press, 1984, Oxford.

Davidson, D (1970a). How is weakness of the will possible? In *Actions and events*, pp. 21–42. Clarendon Press, 1980, Oxford.

Davidson, D (1970b). Mental events. In *Actions and events*, pp. 207–27. Clarendon Press, 1980, Oxford.

Davidson, D (1973). The material mind. In *Actions and events*, pp. 245–59. Clarendon Press, 1980, Oxford.

Davidson, D (1974a). Psychology as philosophy. In *Actions and events*, pp. 229–44. Clarendon Press, 1980, Oxford.

Davidson, D (1974b). Belief and the basis of meaning. In *Truth and interpretation*, pp. 141–54. Clarendon Press, 1980, Oxford.

Davidson, D (1974c). On the very idea of a conceptual scheme. In *Truth and interpretation*, pp. 183–98. Clarendon Press, 1984, Oxford.

Davidson, D (1975). Thought and talk. In *Truth and interpretation*, pp. 155–79. Clarendon Press, 1984, Oxford.

Davidson, D (1978). Intending. In *Actions and events*, pp. 83–102. Clarendon Press, 1980, Oxford.

Davidson, D (1980). *Actions and events*, Clarendon Press, Oxford.

Davidson, D (1982). Paradoxes of irrationality. In R Wolheim and J Hopkins, ed. *Philosophical essays on Freud*, pp. 289–305. Cambridge University Press, Cambridge.

Davidson, D (1984). *Truth and interpretation*, Clarendon Press, Oxford.

Dennett, D (1978). *Brainstorms*, MIT Press, Cambridge MA.

Dennett, D (1987). *The intentional stance*, MIT Press, Cambridge MA.

Edelman, G (1987). *Neural Darwinism*, Basic Books, New York.

Edelson, M (1984). *Hypothesis and evidence in psychoanalysis*, University of Chicago Press, Chicago.

Edelson, M (1988). *Psychoanalysis: a theory in crisis*, University of Chicago Press, Chicago.

Erikson, E (1950). *Childhood and society*, Norton, New York.

Fagen, R (1981). *Animal play behavior*, Oxford University Press, Oxford.

Fishman, J (1993). New clues surface about the making of mind. *Science*, 262, 1517.

Fodor, J (1975). *The language of thought*, Harvard University Press, Cambridge, MA.

Fodor, J (1986). Why paramecia don't have mental representations. *Midwest Studies in Philosophy*, **10**, 3–23.

Franfurt, H (1988). Freedom of the will and the concept of a person. In *The importance of what we care about*, pp.11–25. Cambridge University Press, 1988, Cambridge.

Freud, A (1936). *The ego and the mechanisms of defense*. International Universities Press, 1966, New York.

Freud, A (1981). *Psychoanalytic psychology of normal development*. International Universities Press, New York.

Freud, S (1895). *Project for a scientific psychology*. Standard Edition, Vol. 1. Trans. and ed. J Strachey. Hogarth Press, 1953, London.

Freud, S (1900). *The interpretation of dreams*. Standard Edition, Vol. 4 & 5. Trans. and ed. J Strachey. Hogarth Press, 1953, London.

Freud, S (1905a[1961]). *Fragment of an analysis of a case of hysteria*. Standard Edition, Vol. 7. Trans. and ed. J Strachey. Hogarth Press, 1953, London.

Freud, S (1905b). *Three essays on the theory of sexuality*. Standard Edition, Vol. 7. Trans. and ed. J Strachey. Hogarth Press, 1953, London.

Freud, S (1906[1905]). *My view on the part played by sexuality in the aetiology of the neuroses*. Standard Edition, Vol. 7. Trans. and ed. J Strachey. Hogarth Press, 1953, London.

Freud, S (1907). *Obsessive actions and religious practices*. Standard Edition, Vol. 9. Trans. and ed. J Strachey. Hogarth Press, 1959, London.

Freud, S (1909). *Notes upon a case of obsessional neurosis*. Standard Edition, Vol. 10. Trans. and ed. J Strachey. Hogarth Press, 1955, London.

Freud, S (1913 [1912–13]). *Totem and taboo*. Standard Edition, Vol.13. Trans. and ed. J. Strachey. Hogarth Press, 1957, London.

Freud, S (1915a). *Instincts and their vicissitudes*. Standard Edition, Vol.14. Trans. and ed. J Strachey. Hogarth Press, 1957, London.

Freud, S (1915b). *The unconscious.* Standard Edition, Vol. 14. Trans. and ed. J Strachey. Hogarth Press, 1957, London.

Freud, S (1916). *Some characters met with in psychoanalytic work.* Standard Edition, Vol. 14. Trans. and ed. J Strachey. Hogarth Press, 1957, London.

Freud, S (1917). *A childhood recollection from "Dichtung und Wahrheit".* Standard Edition, Vol. 17. Trans. and ed. J Strachey. Hogarth Press, 1955, London.

Freud, S (1918). *An infantile neurosis.* Standard Edition, Vol. 17. Trans. and ed. J Strachey. Hogarth Press, 1955, London.

Freud, S (1919). *"A child is being beaten": a contribution to the study of the origin of sexual perversions.* Standard Editon, Vol. 17. Trans. and ed. J Strachey. Hogarth Press, 1955, London.

Freud, S (1920). *Beyond the pleasure principle.* The Standard Edition, Vol. 18. Trans. and ed. J Strachey. Hogarth Press, 1955, London.

Freud, S (1926). *Inhibitions symptoms and anxiety.* Standard Edition, Vol. 20. Trans. and ed. J Strachey. Hogarth Press, 1959, London.

Freud, S (1940). *An outline of psycho-analysis.* Standard Edition, Vol. 23. Trans. and ed. J Strachey. Hogarth Press, 1964, London.

Gardner, S (1993). *Irrationality and the philosophy of psychoanalysis,* Cambridge University Press, Cambridge.

Gentner, D (1988). *Metaphor as structure mapping: the relational shift. Child Development,* **58**, 47–59.

Greenberg, M (1972). *Euclidean and non-euclidean geometries: development and history.* W.H. Freeman & Co., New York.

Grunbaum, A (1984). *The foundation of psychoanalysis: a philosophical critique.*University of California Press, Berkeley.

Hursthouse, R (1991). A-rational actions. *Journal of Philosophy,* **88**, 57–68.

Jimenez, L (2002). Surfing on consciousness, or, a deliberately shallow outline of cognition. Commentary on Perruchet and Vinter (2002). The self-organizing consciousness. *Behavioral and Brain Sciences,* **25**, 342.

Kant, I (1781, 1787). *Critique of pure reason.* Trans. Norman Kemp Smith. St. Martin's Press, 1965, New York.

Kant, I (1783). *Prolegomena to any future metaphysics.* ed. and introduced Lewis Beck White. Bobbs-Merrill Co.Inc., 1950, New York.

Keisler, A and Willingham, D (2002). Unconscious abstraction in motor learning. Commentary on Perruchet and Vinter (2002). The self-organizing consciousness. *Behavioral and Brain Sciences,* **25**, 342–3.

Kitcher, P (1990). *Kant's transcendental psychology,* Oxford University Press, New York.

Koffka, K (1925). *The growth of the mind.* Trans. R Ogden. Harcourt, Brace and Co., New York.

Kohler, W (1929). *Gestalt psychology.* Harcourt, Brace and Co., New York.

Lambert, A (2002). The reported demise of the cognitive uncouscious is premature. Commentary on Perruchet and Vinter (2002). The self-organizing consciousness. *Behavioral and Brain Sciences,* **25**, 344–5.

Lear, J (1990). *Love and its place in nature,* Farrar, Strauss and Giroux, New York.

Lear, J (1998). *Open minded,* Harvard University Press, Cambridge MA.

Lewis, D (1988). What experience teaches. In W Lycan, ed. *Mind and cognition: a reader*, pp. 499–519. Blackwell Press, Oxford.

Lorenz, K (1950). The comparative method in studying innate bird behavior patterns. In *Physiological mechanisms in animal behavior*, Symposia of the Society for Experimental Biology. Academic Press, New York.

Millikan, R (1984). *Language, thought, and other biological categories*, MIT Press, Cambridge MA.

Millikan, R (1993). *White queen psychology and other essays for Alice*, MIT Press, Cambridge, MA.

Millikan, R (1993). Thoughts without laws. In *White queen psychology and other essays for Alice*, Chapt. 3, pp. 51–82. MIT Press, Cambridge MA.

Millikan, R (1993). Biosemantics. In *White queen psychology and other essays for Alice*, Chapt 4, pp. 83–101. MIT Press, Cambridge MA,

Millikan, R (1993). On Mentalese orthography. In *White queen psychology and other essays for Alice*, Part 1, Chapt 5, pp. 103–21. MIT Press, Cambridge, MA.

Millikan, R (1993). Explanations in biopsychology. In *White queen psychology and other essays for Alice*. Chapt 9, pp. 172–92. MIT Press, Cambridge, MA.

Moore, B and Fine, B (1990). (eds) *Psychoanalytic terms and concepts*, Yale University Press, New Haven.

McClelland, D and Atkinson, J (1948). The projective expression of needs: I. The effect of different intensities of hunger drive on perception. *Journal of Psychology*, **25**, 205–22.

Murphy, G (1933). *General psychology*, Harper and Brothers, New York and London.

Nagera, H (1969). *Basic psychoanalytic concepts on the libido theory*, Vol. 1. Basic Books, New York.

Nagera, H (1970). *Basic psychoanalytic concepts on the theory of instincts*, Vol. 3. Basic Books, New York.

Novick, J and Novick, K (1996). A developmental perspective on omnipotence. *Journal of Clinical Psychoanalysis*, **5**, 129–73.

Novick, J and Novick, K (2000). Love in the therapeutic alliance. *Journal of the American Psychoanalytic Association*, **48**, 189–218.

Parisse, C and Cohen, H (2002). Oral and visual language are not processed in like fashion. Commentary on Perruchet and Vinter (2002). The self-organizing cousciousness. *Behavioral and Brain Sciences*, **25**, 349–50.

Perruchet, P and Vinter, A (2002). The self-organizing consciousness. *Behavioral and Brain Sciences*, **25**, 297–330.

Poincaire, H (1907). *Science and hypothesis*, The Walter Scott Publishing Co. and Scribner and Sons, London and New York.

Popper, K (1963). *Conjectures and Refutations*, Routledge and Kegan Paul, London.

Rapaport, D (1944a). The scientific methodology of psychoanalysis. In M Gill, ed. *The collected papers of David Rapaport*, pp. 165–220. Basic Books, New York.

Rapaport, D (1957). Psychoanalysis as a developmental psychology. In M Gill, ed. *The collected papers of David Rapaport*, pp. 820–52. Basic Books, 1967, New York.

Rapaport, D (1960). On the psychoanalysis theory of motivation. In M Gill, ed. *The collected papers of David Rapaport*, pp. 853–915. Basic Books, 1967, New York.

Reichenbach, H (1951). *The rise of scientific philosophy*, The University of California Press, Berkeley and Los Angeles.

Reichenbach, H (1958). *The philosophy of space and time*. Trans. M Reichenbach and J Freund. Dover Publications, New York.

Rivera-Gaxiola, M and Silva-Pereyra, J (2002). Is syntax a representation in itself? Commentary on Perruchet and Vinter (2002). The self-organizing consciousness. *Behavioral and Brain Sciences*, **25**, 352–3.

Rubenstein, B (1976). On the possibility of a strictly clinical psychoanalytic theory: an essay in the philosophy of psychoanalysis. In M Gill and P Holzman, ed. *Psychology versus Metapsychology*, pp. 229–64. International Universities Press, New York.

Schroeder, T (2004). *Three faces of desire*, Oxford University Press, Oxford.

Searle, J (1992). *The rediscovery of the mind*, MIT Press, Cambridge MA.

Shevrin, H (1984). The fate of the five metapsychological principles. *Psychoanalytic Inquiry*, **4**, 33–58.

Shevrin, H (1986). A proposed function of consciousness relevant to theory and practice. Presentation, *American Psychological Meetings, Divison 39*, Washington, DC, August 22.

Shevrin, H (1988). The Freud-Rapaport theory of consciousness. in R Bornstein, ed. *Empirical perspectives on the psychoanalytic unconscious*, pp. 45–70. American Psychological Association Press, Washington DC.

Shevrin, H (1995). Is psychoanalysis once science, two sciences, or no science at all? *Journal of the American Psychoanalytic Association*, **43**, 963–86. Commentaries. *Journal of the American Psychoanalytic Association*, **43**, 986–1049.

Shevrin, H (1998). Why do we need consciousness? A psychoanalytic answer. In DF Barone, M Hersen and VB Van Hasselt, ed. *Advanced Personality*, Chapt.10, Plenum Press, New York.

Shevrin, H, Bond J, Hertel, R, Marshall, R,Williams,W, and Brakel, LAW (1992). Event-related potential indicators of the dynamic unconscious. *Consciousness and Cognition*, **1**, 340–66.

Shevrin, H, Bond J, Brakel LAW, Hertel, R, and Williams,W (1996). *Conscious and unconscious processes: psychodynamic, cognitive, and neurophysiologic convergences*, Guilford Press, New York.

Sklar, L (1974). *Space, time and spacetime*, University of California Press, Berkeley and Los Angeles.

Smith, L (1989). From global similarities to kinds of similarities: the construction of Dimension. In S Vosniadou and A Ortony, ed. *Similarity and analogical reasoning*, pp. 146–78. Cambridge University Press, Cambridge.

Snodgrass, M, Shevrin, H, and Kopka, M (1993). The mediation of intentional Judgments by unconscious perceptions: the influences of task strategy, task preference, word meaning, and motivation. *Consciousness and Cognition*, **2**, 194–203.

Spelke, E (1983). *Cognition in Infancy*. Occasional paper No.23, June. MIT Press, Cambridge, MA.

Spelke, E (1990). Principles of object perception. *Cognitive Science*, **14**, 29–56.

Spelke, E and Hermer, L (1996). Early cognitive development: objects and space. In Rochel Gelman and Terry Kit-Fong, ed. *Perceptual and cognitive development*, pp. 71–114. Academic Press, San Diego.

Stampe, D (1987). The authority of desire. *Philosophical Review*, **96**, 335–81.

Stanovich, K and West, R (2001). Individual differences in reasoning: implications for the rationality debate. *Behavioral and Brain Sciences*, **23**, 645–66.

Stich, S (1983). *From folk psychology to cognitive science: the case against belief*, MIT Press, Cambridge, MA.

Stich, S (1990). *The fragmentation of reason*, MIT Press, Cambridge, MA.

Strawson, G (1994). *Mental reality* MIT Press, Cambridge MA.

Symon, R (1978a). *Play and aggression: a study of rhesus monkeys*, Columbia University Press, New York.

Timbergen, N (1951). *The study of instinct*, Clarendon Press, Oxford.

Velleman, JD (1989). *Practical reflection*, Princeton University Press, Princeton, NJ.

Velleman, JD (1998). How belief aims at the truth. Unpublished manuscript.

Velleman, JD (2000). *The possibility of practical reason*, Oxford University Press, Oxford.

Velleman, JD (2002). Motivation by ideal. *Philosophical Explorations*, **5**, 89–104.

Wallerstein, R (1988). One psychoanalysis or many? *International Journal of Psychoanalysis*, **69**, 5–21.

Wallerstein, R (1990). Psychoanalysis: the common ground. *International Journal of Psychoanalysis*, **71**, 3–20.

Wallerstein, R (2005a). Will psychoanalytic pluralism be an enduring state of our discipline? *International Journal of Psychoanalysis*, **86**, 623–6.

Williamson, T (1994). *Vagueness*, Routledge, London and New York.

Wimmer, H and Penner, J (1983). Beliefs about beliefs: representations and constraining functions of wrong belief in young children's understanding of deception. *Cognition*, **13,** 103–28.

Wisdom, J (1953). *Philosophy and psycho-analysis*, University of California Press, Berkeley.

Wolheim, R (1979). Wish fulfillment. In R Harrison, ed. *Rational action*, pp. 47–60. Cambridge University Press, Cambridge.

Wohlheim, R (1984). *The thread of life*, Harvard University Press, Cambridge MA.

Yamauchi, T (2002). The self-organizing consciousness entails additional intervening subsystems. Commentary on Perruchet and Vinter (2002). The self-organizing consciousness. *Behavioral and Brain Sciences*, **25**, 360.

Index

Note: "n." after a page reference indicates the number of a note on that page.